The Brazilian Bikini Body Program

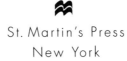

St. Martin's Press
New York

The
BRAZILIAN BIKINI BODY
PROGRAM

30 Days
to a Sexier Body
and Mind

Regina Joseph

www.stmartins.com

Library of Congress Cataloging-in-Publication Data

ISBN-13: 978-0-312-36382-6
ISBN-10: 0-312-36382-6

First Edition: May 2007

10 9 8 7 6 5 4 3 2 1

For my family

Contents

The Brazilian Bikini Body Program

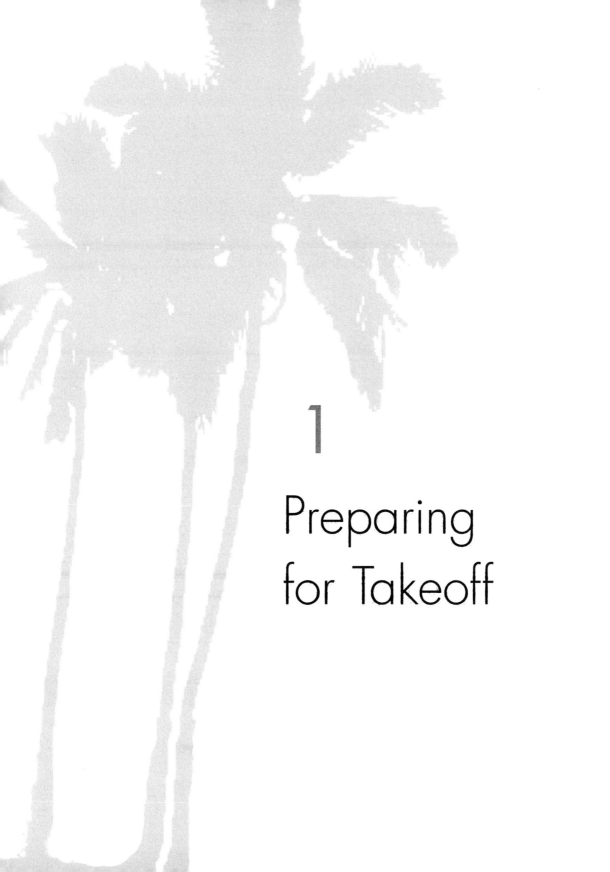

1

Preparing
for Takeoff

I SAT WAITING for my flight from Paris to Rio de Janeiro, when the sight of a fellow passenger became the impetus behind this book.

She was an elegant and lively brunette, chatting animatedly into her mobile phone. Surrounding her were a variety of passengers: some elderly and dignified couples; many French tourists; and even more young women and men, a majority of whom appeared to be attractive teenage Brazilians returning home from Europe.

The brunette stood out. She embodied what has become to many foreigners the cliché of a Brazilian—the girl from Ipanema: tall and tan and young and lovely. She cooed the Brazilian dialect of Portuguese into her phone. As the rapid-fire words tumbled from her mouth, she sprinkled her conversation liberally with affectionate endearments such as *meu querido* ("my darling"), *eu sou sua gatinha* ("I'm your little pussycat"), *meu fofinho* ("my cuddly little one"), and so on.

While I don't normally indulge in eavesdropping, I felt compelled to observe her and her conversation, if only to clarify some of my own thoughts on Brazil and Brazilians. Although I was born in New York City and have lived in Europe and Asia, my parents were born in Brazil, and I've managed over my lifetime to make many visits to relatives and friends in Rio and other locations in Brazil. However, it's only been within the last few years that Brazil's spell has begun to take hold—both on me and on the rest of the world.

I'd never given much thought to what had always been familiar to me. The food I grew up eating; the language I grew up hearing and speaking; the music I listened to and the movies I watched; the art and architecture that formed a big part of my visual education; the movement habits that were second nature; and, most of all, the affectionate exuberance that characterized my experience of other Brazilians—all of these things were brought into focus for me by the vision of this woman at the airport.

This vital, beautiful, happy traveler glowed with good health, a good disposition, and joie de vivre. She represented the ideal to which so many aspire, whether they seek a better body, better health, or a better frame of mind. What woman doesn't want to be the girl from Ipanema? Who, man or woman, doesn't want to approach their lives with a winning smile and a body to match, no matter what the circumstances? It's an attitude, a look, and a presence that I call the Brazilian Bikini Body, and I'm going to show you how to get it.

The Brazilian Bikini Body Program, or BBBP, is a holistic system that addresses

TEN SIMPLE BRAZILIAN PHRASES YOU SHOULD KNOW

1. What's up? = *Aí galera* [ay-EE ga-LEH-rah]
2. Cool = *Legal* [leh-GOWL], *sinistro* [see-NEE-stroo], *manera* [mah-NEH-rah] (synonyms)
3. Delicious = *Gostoso* [go-SHTOH-zoo]
4. Beautiful woman = *Gostosa* [go-SHTOH-za], *gata* [GAH-tah] (means "cat")
5. Beautiful man = *Bonitão* [boh-nee-TUNH], *gato* [GAH-too]
6. Thanks! = *Valeu!* [vah-LEU]
7. Not my cup of tea = *Não e minha praia* [nunh eh MEE-nyah pry-ah] (means "it's not my beach")
8. Dude! = *Cara!* [KAH-ra]
9. Kisses and hugs = *Beijos e abraços* [BEH-zhoos ee ah-BRAH-soos]
10. Religion = *Futebol* [FOO-chee-bawl]

both body and mind in three parts: attitude, food, and movement. It is based on Brazilian foods, culture, and, most important, style. By following it, you can sculpt a body fit for the beach in Rio, and adopt an outlook resilient enough to shrug off whatever life throws at you, as well as the flair to carry it off memorably. The BBBP asks you to use panache in investing in yourself as a whole person as opposed to using inhuman discipline to squeeze yourself into a microscopic bathing suit. To Brazilians, *boa vida*, or the good life, rests on food, festivity, and fun. We all have the same limitations—time, money, and energy—but a fun program makes it much easier to reorganize your life. The BBBP will steer you away from denial and discomfort, and toward efficient, enjoyable food and play.

If you have ever dieted before, you know that it is all but impossible to stay longterm on a restricted meal plan and keep the weight off. And, as study after study has shown, a program of caloric deprivation without some kind of exercise will only make the inevitable rebound weight gain worse . . . and more difficult to lose again.

How do the Brazilians do it? They don't deprive themselves, or beat themselves up at the gym, and yet they radiate vitality and embrace life. The answer lies in attitude. Brazilians view eating as an opportunity to savor delicious and nutritious meals in the midst of their busy lives. Second, they include movement—fun, playful movement—as part of their everyday experience.

The Brazilian Bikini Body Program

Another secret, maybe more important than the first two, is in the very spirit of Brazil, a nation of people who are renowned for their vivacity, passion, and openness—in spite of the obstacles they face. It is this quality of cheerful gusto, despite vast problems, that the Brazilian Bikini Body Program will give you.

The key to this positive outlook is *jeito* [ZHAY-too], Portuguese for "way" or "manner." Often a diminuitive suffix is added to create the colloquial *jeitinho*, [zhay-CHEE-nyoo], which means "that special little way" or "that little knack."

For a Brazilian, the *jeitinho* principally refers to how one gets around any snafu. The *jeitinho* is the soul of flexibility and as such can accommodate as wide a range of actions as possible. It can encompass how a meal is served; to how a soccer ball is kicked; to how one treats one's friends, clients, or guests. Brazilians employ a unique *jeitinho* that blends pragmatism, cheeky irreverence, sometimes ruthlessness, humor, and lust for life into a compelling national comportment that foreigners can easily identify. It's what makes the Brazilian Carnival so much more epic and fun than other countries' pre-Lenten displays; it's what makes soccer fanatics root for Brazil no matter where they come from; it's why people who visit Brazil tend to come back again and again. The Brazilian *jeitinho*, once experienced, gets under the skin.

Get the Knack

Tem jeito?

These two little words form a question that embodies the very heart of Brazilian life. Translated as, "Is there a way around things?" the query—occasionally uttered in a low whisper while furtively glancing around to ensure no one's listening—pops up in every conceivable situation requiring an expedient solution.

Jeito represents the ultimate weapon Brazilians use to confront the miasma of bureaucracy, corruption, and inefficiency that they may endure on a daily basis. Finding an end run around impossibly difficult circumstances has even become a cottage industry in Brazil. Every city and town in Brazil has its corps of *despachantes* (loosely translated as "accelerators"), professional fixers whose job it is to use their resources of connections, influence, and sometimes bribes and favors to cut through red tape—for a fee, of course.

Brazil has shuddered through waves of political instability and military dictatorship to find itself saddled with a distended government and byzantine civil service structure that can make everyday life trying. In a quest to obtain any basic required document, such as a passport, driver's license, or national identity card, the average person usually suffers obscenely long waits and catch-22 barriers. So citizens turn to the *despachantes* to *dar um jeitinho* ("sort it out").

The *jeitinho* does not always stay on the right side of the law. Indeed, the term *jeitinho* conjures shades of illegality, even criminality—mostly due to the long history of politicians and the rich employing *jeitinhos* among cronies to enhance their power and wealth at the expense of a poorer majority. Brazilians have become accustomed to a familiar slogan regarding their politicians: *Rouba, mas faz* ("He steals, but gets things done"). But it's not only bigwigs who use questionable *jeitinhos*. Riding in a taxi in downtown Rio one day, I got stuck in choking traffic on my way back to Ipanema. The driver could see I was fidgeting—I was going to be late for an appointment—and said, "*Não se preoccupe, vou dar um jeitinho*," ("Don't you worry, I'll sort it out"). He then proceeded to drive over the street barrier onto the other lane, got off on a side street, and then gleefully ran through four red lights as if he was Ayrton Senna—the Brazilian Formula 1 champion—until we arrived at my destination. I arrived on time.

Jeitinho is not all bad. At its core, the notion of *jeitinho* extends to any basic coping mechanism that makes life easier. It can be deployed without breaking any laws or rules to achieve welcome ends, such as helping a friend out; protecting your family; or improving your outlook on a tricky matter.

Consider the necessity for pragmatism and self-effacing humor among Brazilians: In 2004, the public debt accounted for 52 percent of the country's gross domestic product; the currency has changed and fluctuated for decades; one-fifth of the population lives below the poverty line and routinely goes hungry. Yet, Brazil is one of the world's largest producers and exporters of meat, grain, and fruit, as well as such critical resources as oil, cotton, and iron ore. It's the fifth largest country in the world and yet it does not have a centralized rail network to effectively cover the immensity of its geographical span (Brazilians sarcastically refer to their rail system as "the road option"). In 2002, the country elected Luiz Inacio da Silva—otherwise known in affectionate Brazilian shorthand as Lula—as president. A former Marxist and pleb fist-shaker, he came to power on thundered promises of zero corruption, only to watch three years later as all his fellow Worker's Party cronies and cabinet ministers came undone in a farcical explosion of bribe-taking and misappropriation of funds. Indeed, life in Brazil is a paradox that tests the patience of its citizens mightily. It is a paradise of extraordinary bounty and beauty that has shocking levels of bureaucracy, crime, and misery. And yet, the essence of the Brazilian *jeitinho* is to lead one's life with as much pleasure and fun as one can, in spite of the enormous obstacles that present themselves. If you can find a way to humorously mock the travails that are beyond your power to control, then you've gotten the Brazilian *jeitinho* just right.

The Brazilian Bikini Body Program

With the BBBP, I'd like to reclaim the positive value of the *jeitinho* and put it to use. Everyone knows that changing your life by managing your diet and exercise takes great effort. Sometimes it feels so overwhelming, and the urge to quit is so strong, that caving in occurs relatively early in the process. Success in sticking with it requires some mental readjustments, so here's where the notion of *jeitinho* comes into play.

The lucky denizens of such gorgeous locales as Rio and Salvador know that when the going gets tough, they can go to the beach, because at least it's free. And if you can't get to the beach, having a stroll and a nice *cafezinho* (coffee served strong, black, and in a small portion, like a shot) while taking a moment to admire the weather or the sensuous figures of passersby is just as much a facet of the *jeitinho*. Food, and the pleasure of eating and savoring it, also account for a large part of *jeitinho*. In Brazil, people eat three distinct meals during the day and plan their activities around meals, emphasizing food's importance. Outside mealtimes, people are in constant motion, whether for work or for leisure. If you can incorporate these building blocks into your daily routine, you'll have found the *jeitinho* for yourself.

You may find yourself saying, "But that's easier said than done. I work at least twelve hours a day, I've got kids to take care of, I've got too many bills to pay, I've got too many demands on my time." Of course you do. Time is always a threat to a well-intentioned *jeitinho*. But to that end, I've developed the program in such a way that the meal plan emphasizes a majority of recipes that can be prepared quickly, easily, and cheaply. The movement component of the program involves both short and long routines to suit your availability of time, but, in its own *jeitinho*, emphasizes doing whatever you can if you can't manage or bear either routine

By learning how to be like the women and men who walk along the beaches of Rio de Janeiro, clad in skimpy *tangas* or *fio dental* (dental floss) and *sunga* swimwear, happy to show their bodies, whether skinny or robust; all of them eating, playing, and most of all laughing; ultimately, anyone can glow like that woman I saw in Paris that night on my way back to Brazil.

You Can't Force What Does Not Want to Be Forced

For a long time, I rejected much of the wisdom passed down to me, especially when it came to the lessons my father was eager to impart.

Having grown up in Ipanema, my father was very athletic. Cariocas, or Brazilians from Rio de Janeiro, are a health-oriented and sporty bunch who are constantly on the move. My father was raised playing soccer, swimming, running, and doing calisthenics. My earliest memories are of his doing tricks with a soccer ball and encouraging me to capture the ball from him by using footwork.

As a child, I did not fit his athletic ideal. A defiant tomboy, I was obsessed with skateboarding (I toted a little banana yellow deck virtually everywhere I went), horse-back riding, swimming, and body-boarding/surfing. Still, I had a tendency toward puppy fat.

My father saw me as a rebellious lazybones and tried to remedy my failing by in-stilling in me an appreciation for daily exercise sessions. He demonstrated countless sit-ups, push-ups, and stretches on the floor of our living room and then insisted that I do the same with him watching over me. I hated the sessions, but not quite as much as I hated my father's lecturing me on exercise.

His intentions were good, although his method of delivery lacked finesse. He knew what many instinctively understand but do not practice: Being healthy is a primary component of happiness, and to remain healthy you must eat well and stay active throughout your life. But whether you are a smart-mouthed kid who'd rather listen to music than do fifty push-ups, or an adult leading a hectic life and having difficulty find-ing time and energy for a workout, the bottom line is this: You cannot force what does not want to be forced.

Ultimately, the desire to be active has to be self-motivated, whether it comes from a personal epiphany about maintaining your health or, more important, having positive experiences when exercising which, in turn, create a habit of it.

Despite my distaste for my father's daily calisthenics sessions, which had all the charm of the Bataan Death March as far as my young mind was concerned, my atten-tion turned to team sports when I became a teenager. I was never a truly great athlete, but that didn't stop me from working hard. As I got older and work took over from aca-demia, my life became an ambitious quest for success and creative innovation. I became a journalist and media developer, structuring my life around deadlines and projects. Proper eating habits and activity fell by the wayside. I watched as my weight yo-yoed up and down, and at one point, my only fuel was cigarettes and Chinese takeout. I devel-oped a rapid heartbeat and wound up having to go to a cardiologist. Being resilient and young, I shook off the dizziness and heart palpitations and resolved to quit smoking when I turned thirty. Around the same time, I took up Pilates, a concession I made to finally dealing with the lower back pain that all my computer work was causing.

I surged forward in the corporate rat race, and my workloads became ever more stressful. I was maintaining households in Europe and Manhattan, commuting between offices in Amsterdam and London on a weekly basis and regularly flying to Japan, San

Francisco, Scandinavia, and South America. I struggled to eat well and do Pilates a couple of times a week—the one thing that managed to keep me alive. My hectic schedule was having an effect: My body was beginning to break down. My hair began to fall out, colds never seemed to completely go away, my gastrointestinal system was a mess, and I was a walking zombie due to insomnia. Changing time zones weekly, eating junky snacks and bad airplane and hotel food, coping with interminable meetings, and the stress of dealing with the ghastly politics of the media business all combined to yield a frightening diagnosis: adrenal fatigue. A frank discussion with my doctor confirmed a long-held, nagging suspicion: If I didn't quit what I was doing soon and orient my life toward a healthier and less stressful path, I wasn't going to have much life left.

As scary as that prognosis was, it was nowhere near as scary as the changes it would require. If I quit work that paid me extremely handsomely, how could I keep my lifestyle going? In the end, I reasoned, a life with less stuff is better than no life at all. After all, I was fortunate and had more than any person could reasonably need. I came up with a plan that put my well-being first, knowing intuitively that if I managed to turn that around, everything else would fall into place.

I resolved to get out of the corporate media world and become certified as a Pilates instructor. I took two years off, focusing on nothing other than my certifications, studying anatomy, biomechanics, kinesiology, and nutrition. I was working out daily; cooking balanced meals based on, among other things, the Brazilian recipes of my childhood; and taking my dog for long walks. I was living off my savings, which meant that I was on an austerity plan that required monkish devotion to frugality. I also knew that for at least a few years, any work I got would yield far less than a starting salary for a college graduate.

Despite the stress of downsizing my life, my overall happiness was increasing exponentially. I gradually regained my mental and physical health. I eventually opened up my own Pilates studio as well as a well-being consultancy, and I returned to freelance magazine writing. Slowly but surely, it began to pay off.

I've watched my life come full circle. The irony is rich; after resisting my father's entreaties to follow his lifestyle of daily activity and reasonable eating habits, I've grown up to not only do just that, but to also impart that same advice to others.

The Brazilian Bikini Body Program promotes the concept of doing what you can, without guilt, without feeling pushed, with only the constant and gentle reminder that anything you can manage is better than nothing and to take heart in that—it's the first step in your pragmatic journey of living.

The Bounty of Brazil

Those of us lucky enough to be in a position where we have so much food or luxury time to enjoy that we need to find ways of reducing the bulk or unhealthy habits we've acquired, are the fortuitous "haves." Believe it or not, what we eat and how we eat have massive ramifications for Brazil and for the world in general. Moreover, we should spare a thought for the state of the "have-nots," the people whose lives our consumption directly affects.

The Amazon rainforest has been called the Earth's "lungs," as it is the largest rainforested region on earth, covering a landmass almost the same size as the continental United States. In the last three decades, one-fifth (approximately 204,000 square miles) of the rainforest has been cleared to provide land for cattle ranching for cheap meat production and arable soil for soybean farming.

A love for Brazil and its incredible resources is implicitly tied to a love for the rainforest. So many of Brazil's most delicious and nutritious foods come from the forest. Without the forest and its unmatched biodiversity, many of the modern medicines we use, as well as the cures we hope for in the future, would not exist. Most important, the more reduced the forest, the greater the greenhouse effect. The huge green mass that is the rainforest breathes in the carbon spewed by our industrialized society, and breathes out oxygen. Already, our planet is overwhelmed with too much carbon dioxide. Clearing the forest for more fields, more ranches, or more housing only makes matters worse by destroying the Earth's natural protections. By ignoring what we do today, we create trouble for tomorrow.

With the BBBP, you have a chance to change yourself and the world at the same time. Buying some of the products required in the BBBP's eating plan—specifically the *açaí* fruit that is a cornerstone of each day's menu—can aid the reforestation of the Amazon. By supporting production and harvesting of indigenous plants like *açaí* palms among the small mom-and-pop subsistence farming communities in the Amazon, the land becomes more profitable through cultivation of *açaí*, rather than beef ranching, which requires cutting and clearing trees. The incentive not only to keep indigenous Amazonian trees but plant new ones becomes more compelling—and all the more pressing—as the rapid rate of deforestation has already begun to create severe water shortages in formerly lush Amazonian states, such as Acre.

In addition, Amazonian farmers are often poor and lack clout; they present a stark contrast to our privileged lives. But when buying *açaí* and other Brazilian products (such as nuts and fruits) through reputable companies that comply with fair trade programs designed to improve the living conditions of people who organically harvest the rainforest's plants, we are doing something good for our bodies, for the Earth, and for people whose lives are so very different from our own. Compassion and respect for others and for nature is the foundation for a real Brazilian *jeitinho*.

I am not a doctor, and I stress that the program is not a treatment or a "cure." However, as a well-being professional, my job being to teach and encourage people to maximize their existing strengths, I suggest that the BBBP is a cultural interpretation of some fairly basic and obvious truths: (1) Eat Earth-friendly, tasty foods that are good for you, and allow yourself the occasional indulgence; (2) stay active, even if that means a quick run around the block, since anything is better than nothing at all; and (3) be kind, open, and enjoy what you're doing, especially this program. Put on a bikini or swimming trunks, dance around the house with a bossa nova blaring, and don't be afraid to have a little goofy fun. Be seductive, be playful, don't be afraid. Just take a look at photos of all the bejeweled old grandmas, plump cuties, and perfect-bodied, cat-like teens waving and dancing the samba on Carnival floats. They couldn't care less about wrinkles, bumps, lumps, or problems. For a period of time, they experience only what gives them and those around them happiness. Emulating that makes for good exercise. Finally, never take yourself or this program too seriously. Laughing at yourself is excellent therapy, in addition to being good for your abs.

Moving Forward

In three basic steps, the BBBP can help you reorient your life toward a smarter and healthier path. The internal changes that these steps will precipitate will eventually make themselves manifest externally.

The noted natural attractiveness of Brazil's citizens (and their ability to maintain their good looks throughout their long lives) exists for two important reasons. One is genetic, as Brazil has become throughout its five-hundred-year history the world's most miscegenated pool of ethnicities, resulting in a legendarily beautiful mélange. The second comes down to the lifestyle which I encourage you to adopt: Brazilians eat fruits, vegetables, grains, fish, and meat that are extremely rich in nutrients; they are constantly outdoors and active; and they strive to stay up even when life gets them down. This is the core of the Brazilian Bikini Body Program. Follow it, and you, too, will experience an increase in your energy, health, and contentedness.

Like anyone else around the world, Brazilians may be bound to the TV when their favorite soap operas commence (known in Portuguese as *novelas*), but apart from work and *novelas*, Brazilians are out and about trying to enjoy their lives.

For the next thirty days, try living the Brazilian Bikini Body Program lifestyle and *fique numa boa* ("stay cool"). It's not as hard as you think. As Brazilians say: *Vamos la!* ("Let's go!")

The Brazilian Bikini Body Program

Attitude

So far, I've talked about the *jeitinho*, or that special little way the BBBP provides for people who want to improve their health. Certainly the food suggestions and movement embody a healthy, Brazilian flair, but where *jeitinho* really comes into its own is in the outlook.

The first objective in this psychic readjustment? Relax. Let go of, as much as possible, your negative and guilty thoughts regarding food and exercise. Brazilians are proud of their laid-back reputation, but that's not to say they are all reckless and carefree. Quite the contrary. Brazilians are simply constitutionally opposed to wasting energy on thoughts and motivations that will not advance them to a more positive position.

Unfortunately, many of our attitudes toward food and activity are colored by a guilt-ridden denial-binge-purge cycle. We avoid eating what we really want until we can stand it no longer; then we go on a hell-bent spree of indulgence, usually followed by shame and a burst of furious, short-lived activity. Then we lapse back into the vicious circle of inactivity, followed by another round of denial-binge-purge.

This book promotes health not skinniness, strength not six-packs. You will lose weight and get toned, but these surface traits should be secondary to your overall vigor. The BBBP encourages practitioners to drop their body image hang-ups by accepting the good as well as the bad about themselves. Brazil may be famous for the vanity of its citizens, but, paradoxically, that self-regard is benevolent in that it encompasses as wide a continuum of shapes and sizes as possible. Bodily perfection is attainable by only a few, and even then, only for a limited time. So why not focus instead on a steady and measured pace that you can enjoy and keep over the long-term?

But it's not enough to be kind to yourself. The BBBP's attitude adjustment integrates an important social consciousness. Food has implications beyond what it does to your body. It has political, societal, and environmental repercussions, too. The fact that some of the BBBP's food products originate from a region in danger provides an opportunity for individuals to extend their desire for improvement beyond themselves toward a wider world.

Food

As Brazilians well know, three good meals a day is an essential part of *boa vida*, the good life. To them, a diet doesn't require deprivation but a sensible approach to delicious food. In that spirit, the BBBP features an eating plan that will never get boring. Its foundation lies in tasty variety based on Brazilian cuisine, moderate portions, and most important, key Brazilian food products rich in nutritional benefits. The BBBP employs the delicious benefits of such Amazonian fruits as the *açaí*, acerola, and coconut, as well as the Brazil nut and the cashew, among many others.

On the global stage of food production, Brazil is the star under the spotlight. It is currently the world's largest agricultural superpower. The country is now the number one exporter of such commodities as orange juice, chicken, coffee, and sugar (as well as other noncomestible exports like iron ore and biofuel). But thanks to its emerging status as the new breadbasket of the Earth, Brazil's more obscure food products, especially the incredible produce from the Amazon, are now becoming more widely and cheaply available to people outside the country. In the last three years, products that never before were seen outside Brazil's local markets are suddenly appearing in your corner store; your local health food and juice bars; your cosmetics counter; and your gym. The BBBP will teach you how to make use of this abundance, as well as explain how it can benefit you.

In addition to presenting a diet and menu plan that capitalizes on the arrival of mouthwatering produce to these shores, the BBBP emphasizes a routine that fits busy lifestyles. One of the biggest obstacles to healthy nutrition is time, and I've designed the diet so that the majority of your meals can be prepared with a minimum of fuss and expense. In particular, breakfast, the most important meal of the day and the one that most people avoid, can now be as easy as pouring milk into cold cereal—but far more appetizing and nutritious. The BBBP provides carbohydrates, proteins, fats, and sugars with no sanctions other than reasonable portion size. You'll look forward to eating.

Movement

The BBBP merges the core strengthening power of Pilates with cardiovascular accents taken from capoeira, the Brazilian martial art.

In Brazil, a tropical country where people spend as much time outdoors as possible, exercise comes naturally. Beach activities like surfing, swimming, volleyball and soccer (and the unique Brazilian hybrid of the two, *fut-volei*), and running and walking are popular. But to maintain the kind of core strength required to excel at these activities (and the kind of shapely bottom that looks good in a *tanga* or thong), Brazilians have elevated Pilates into one of the country's fastest-growing pursuits. A walk along the major streets of such cities as Rio de Janeiro and São Paulo turns up even more Pilates studios than can be found in New York—the city where Joseph Pilates, the German originator of the method, built his studio in 1926.

Add to Pilates the challenging movements of capoeira, a discipline dating back to Brazil's colonial days. Originally created by African slaves as a form of self-defense and a way of resolving disputes among themselves, this deceptive martial art looks like dancing but is fast and deadly when performed well. While the defensive aspect is still taught and used by Brazil's poorest and most disenfranchised citizens, the agility and cardiovascular benefits of capoeira have created a resurgence of popularity among those seeking a fitness alternative both within Brazil and beyond.

Pilates and capoeira have been combined in the BBBP to create interesting and efficient workouts that will strengthen your abdominals and lower-body muscles; increase your balance and stability; reduce postural problems; and improve concentration so that a harmonious mind-body connection can be achieved.

The BBBP offers three workout routines based on varying lengths of time: (1) The Full-Hour Workout consists of a one-hour routine that requires nothing more than a mat and a level floor; (2) the Half-Hour Workout can be completed in about thirty minutes and is designed for optimal fat-burning; and (3) the Mini Workout, a ten-minute routine, can be done virtually anywhere and is perfect for days when you are simply too busy to squeeze in a longer workout. Because the BBBP emphasizes movement whenever and however you can manage, it accounts for those days when you know you won't be able to put time into full exercise sessions.

These three building blocks taken together create something greater than what we've traditionally come to know as "diets." I've never met anybody who actually enjoys dieting. I've certainly gritted my teeth through a few weeks' worth of meal torture, only to find that my willpower eventually caves in after being suffocated for a few weeks with constant denial. The Brazilian Bikini Body Program is an antidiet: The goal is to eat, move, and live mindfully. The benefits will follow.

2

Brazilian Food

BRAZILIAN CUISINE is a mixture of bold flavors created from simple and simply prepared ingredients, many of which are nutritionally potent "superfoods." Certain regional aspects of the cuisine can be quite spicy but, overall, the food is highly seasoned rather than tongue-burning hot.

In the same way that certain cuisines at their most basic level can be generally identified by flavor trinities—Italian food tastes of tomato, garlic, and basil; French food tastes of butter, garlic, and wine; Japanese food tastes of soy sauce, mirin, and dashi; etc.—Brazilian food can be identified by a couple of distinct flavor groups.

The most predominant note comes in the trinity of the aromatics garlic, onion, and bay leaf. What basil is to Italian and southern French food, the bay leaf is to Brazilian food. Its uniquely bracing, arboreal scent underscores the more familiar aroma of garlic and onion, elevating the three notes together to a distinctly memorable smell and taste.

After the aromatics reach the nose, the tongue tastes the second identifiable flavor trinity: astringents. In the case of Brazilian cuisine, the acidic qualities of lime, tomato, and vinegar (or wine) blend and balance against the mildly nutty, vegetal flavors of the olive and *dendê* oils, in which most food is cooked. The very Brazilian combination of aromatic and astringent flavors can be most widely experienced in *vinha d'alho* (Garlic-Wine Marinade, see recipe on page 76), the basic marinade that most meats and fish steep in before cooking.

These flavors support a wide array of meat, fish, vegetables, legumes, and even fruit. But a couple of ingredients figure more heavily than others in the Brazilian diet. For a start, Brazilians are major carnivores. Red meat, in the form of steak, supplies a big part of the protein in the diet. Luckily, Brazilians have high-quality, well-seasoned beef—a fact that draws avid worshippers at the many altars of barbecue. While others may worry about the cardiac implications of consuming so much meat, in general, Brazilians tend to eat very lean cuts and small fillet portions. The BBBP features red meat, but you can substitute good ultra-lean beef alternatives such as buffalo and ostrich, both now becoming more widely available at organic markets. Vegetarians or those watching their cholesterol intake can use chicken, turkey, or soy-based meat substitutes in many of the red-meat recipes in the program.

Seafood, of course, is another prominent component of Brazilian cuisine. Shrimp especially, whether fresh or dried, appears in everything from pies to soups, stews, fritters, sauces and more. Shrimp is an excellent source of lean protein with less of the heavy-metal toxins that unfortunately now make eating some large fish a bit of Russian roulette. Buy frozen shrimp, which can be found at reasonable prices—especially in Asian markets.

Fruits and nuts—especially indigenous Brazilian varieties—feature heavily in both sweet and savory preparations. Dark leafy greens, and legumes such as beans and seeds, round out the country's colorful cuisine, adding diversity and nutrition to the most basic of meals.

This combination of flavors and ingredients provides the key to the Brazilian-based eating plan's success. It's tasty as well as good for you—two important factors that will help you stick to the program.

Brazilian Superfood Pantry Staples

Açaí [ah-SIGH-ee]
While Brazilians generally prefer to eat *açaí* at their favorite local juice bar or on the beach, most supermarkets carry packets of frozen *açaí* to keep in the freezer at home. About four years ago, frozen Brazilian *açaí* pulp was introduced into the American marketplace, and you can now buy it at such stores as Whole Foods. American drinks manufacturers, noting the health benefits of the berry, have rushed to add *açaí* to their juice and smoothie formulations. While any addition of *açaí* to a drink or smoothie will lend its characteristic chocolatey taste, seek frozen preparations where the pulp has not been pasteurized or cooked at high heat, because this destroys most of the berry's nutritional value. Cook with any type of commercial preparation of *açaí* to impart a fantastic berry flavor to savory stews, sweet puddings, and drinks. See page 37 for more about *açaí*.

Acerola [ah-seh-RAW-la], a.k.a. *Cereja de Pará* [seh-REH-zha jee pah-RAH] or Barbados Cherry
When Brazilians start to feel under the weather, many reach for a drink with acerola. This tart fruit with a flavor somewhere between a cherry and an orange is one of the world's richest sources of vitamin C. Three acerola cherries constitute a full day's dosage of vitamin C for the average adult. Commercial preparations of frozen acerola pulp are now available in the United States, but Vitamin C supplements made from acerola have been around for several years now. Studies of acerola supplements and powders have not yielded conclusive results on their efficacy, so you're far better off trying to eat it in its frozen fruit pulp form. Some people simply cut the plastic off the

packages and suck on it like a Popsicle, which makes it easier, more fun, and more nutritious than juicing several oranges to delay an oncoming cold or flu. In addition to using acerola for smoothies and juices, it can be incorporated into refreshing, cold fruit soups.

Bay Leaf, a.k.a. *Folha de Louro* [FOH-lya jee LOH-row]

Greeks and Romans revered this Asian native plant, prizing it as a symbol of honor and glory. For medicinal purposes, bay leaves served as the primary ingredient of applications ranging from insecticides to abortifacients. Ulcers, gastrointestinal disorders, infections, and headaches were all treated with poultices made from the oil of this pungent leaf whose active ingredient, eugenol, has anti-inflammatory properties. It has even been used in the treatment of diabetes: The plant helps lower blood sugar levels by assisting the body's efficient production of insulin. The Portuguese brought the bay leaf to Brazil, most likely through their association with India, one of the bay leaf's native countries. Since adopted into Brazilian cuisine, the bay leaf now serves as one of its predominant flavors. The foundation marinade behind Brazilian cuisine, *vinha d'alho* (see recipe on page 76), should be redolent of bay leaf for authenticity.

Beans, a.k.a. *Feijão* [fay-ZHAO]

Beans and legumes of many varieties form a critical cornerstone of Brazilian cuisine, especially in *feijoada* (see recipe on page 123), the national dish of Brazil that features smoked meats stewed in black beans. But legumes ranging from black-eyed peas (used in the popular fritter known as *acarajé*—see recipe on page 100), to lentils to chickpeas to soybeans all feature widely in the continuum of Brazilian food. Beans are ideal for those seeking a method to help curb hunger and unchecked appetite. The balance of slow-release, complex carbohydrate fuel, fiber, and iron that beans provide guarantee great dishes for dieters that can be prepared quickly and cheaply. Even if you're not watching your weight, the high vitamin, mineral, and fiber content of beans may assist in lowering cholesterol levels and keeping the digestive system in good health.

Brazil Nuts and Cashew Nuts, a.k.a. *Castanha-do-Pará* [kah-SHTUN-yah do pah-RAH] or *Castanha-do-Brasil* (Brazil nut), *Castanha de Caju* (cashew)

Nuts serve many uses in the Brazilian kitchen. They make delicious and easy snacks, but they also act as thickening and flavoring agents, butters and flour. Whether you're in Rio or Fortaleza, you'll often see men casually walking with giant three-foot bags of cashews or peanuts hoisted on their shoulders. Cashews, a Brazilian native plant, uniquely marry two products in one: The fruit of the cashew yields the familiar sweet and chewy nut; attached to the nut fruit is a peduncle that looks like an orange bell pepper. Known as the cashew apple, the peduncle has a sweet, tart, and mouth-puckering apple-like flavor that is beloved in Brazil for use in juices, smoothies, puddings, and just about anything sweet.

The Brazil nut is a classic superfood and the seed of one of the Brazilian rainforest's most majestic trees—many of which reach over 150 feet in height. The nut is a prized and valuable resource. Just two of these meaty nuts contain as much protein as one egg. They are excellent sources of vitamins A, B, and C, and minerals like calcium, phosphorus, and magnesium. The soothing oil of the Brazil nut is used to make not only food but also minimally processed cosmetics with purported health benefits (cosmeceuticals). The WWF, formerly known as World Wildlife Fund, actively supports the trade and marketing of Brazil nut eco-harvesting as a force in preserving the Brazilian rainforest.

Coriander, a.k.a. *Coentro* [koh-EN-troh] or Cilantro

A Mediterranean native plant, coriander appears in many Brazilian savory dishes. Americans usually recognize the fragrant, earthy aroma and taste of coriander from its use in Asian and Mexican cuisines. In Brazil, cooks like to pair coriander with parsley and onion to make *cheiro verde* (Green Aroma—see recipe on page 77) a common flavoring and garnish. Outside of the kitchen, records dating as far back as the Egyptian period note coriander's myriad medicinal properties—such as relief of digestive upsets and inflammation. Once, while traveling on a boat in a severe storm, I suffered extreme nausea. The woman in charge of the kitchen prepared a tea of coriander leaves and seeds and, within ten minutes, I was feeling fine.

Coconut, a.k.a. *Coco* [KOH-koo]

Fewer drinks are more lovely, wholesome, or refreshingly nutritious than an ice-cold green coconut cracked open by a machete and penetrated by a straw. Beach snack kiosks along the entire coast of Brazil decorate their sides with the intact spathes of the coconut palm, bulging with their bounty of emerald globes. Brazilians prize the young, or green, coconut for its water and pulp. The lightly sweet water, rich in vitamins, potassium, and other electrolytes, tastes only mildly of coconut. For years, Brazilian athletes have downed coconut water rather than plain water as a mineral replacement drink during exercising. Kiosks often advertise the benefits of coconut water with signs declaring "*Coco—Saude Gelada*" ("Coconut—Icy-Cold Health"), aimed at runners, surfers, skateboarders, or thirsty strollers. The gelatinous meat inside the coconut can be scraped out—usually with a shard of the coconut that the vendor obligingly hacks off with a machete—once you've finished the water, making this superfood-in-a-versatile-package thirst quenching, delicious, and recyclable. For those who can't get to the beach, fresh coconut-water dispensing carts wind their way through the city streets of Brazil. Older coconuts yield coconut milk (the liquid that results from passing water through the meat of the coconut) and the opaque shreds we typically recognize as shredded coconut. Coconut meat and milk are in many aspects of Brazilian cuisine from savory Bahian seafood stews to sweet puddings, cakes, candies, and cocktails. Processed coconuts also provide the base for an enormous industry in food oils, fuel oils, and cosmetic oils.

Dendê [den-DEH], a.k.a. Red Palm Oil

Captured slaves brought to Brazil over four hundred years ago were responsible for integrating this African native palm and fruit into the culture, botany, and cuisine of Brazil. The unctuous fruit flesh of the *dendê* palm continues to be rendered today into *dendê* oil—not to be confused with the harmful palm kernel oil, which is made from the seed of the *dendê* fruit and which does not have the beneficial properties of *dendê* oil. Like so many other palm products, *dendê* oil's unique taste and versatility in Brazilian cuisine overshadow its important nutritional values. *Dendê* oil, when minimally processed, retains large amounts of vitamin A, which gives it it's characteristically intense crimson-orange color. It also contains vitamin E and linoleic acid, an important omega-6 essential fatty acid that the body requires to heal wounds and keep the hair, skin, and nails healthy. *Dendê* oil, unlike hydrogenated oils that raise cholesterol and contain trans fats, may actually lower harmful LDL cholesterol and inhibit tumor growth, thanks to its powerful carotenoid and tocopherol antioxidants. *Dendê* oil remains solid at room temperature and does not go rancid easily, which makes it a very stable oil to cook with in a tropical climate. For non-equatorial dwellers concerned about the level of saturated fat, *dendê* contains about 40 to 50 percent saturated fat, comparable to an equal amount of butter. Aside from its benefits, *dendê* tastes smooth and nutty, lending an unmistakable flavor and color to the Afro-Brazilian cuisine of Bahia, on the northeastern coast of Brazil. Be careful: Some people's stomachs can be sensitive to *dendê*. If you've never eaten it before, go easy on your first sampling to ensure that you don't develop a stomachache. Once the body is acclimated, however, any digestive upset usually subsides completely.

Garlic, a.k.a. *Alho* [AH-lyoo]

Some people believe that all food tastes better with a little garlic. In the case of Brazilians, make that a lot of garlic. Savory dishes usually involve sautéing garlic and onion before all other ingredients are added. Although garlic's intense flavor and aroma shouldn't eclipse the other flavors of a dish, some Brazilians love it so much that they prefer their garlic unadulterated; I know a few who wouldn't blink twice at the notion of having for breakfast a few slices of toast liberally rubbed with roasted garlic. Garlic serves as a base for Brazilian cuisine's most important marinade, *vinha d'alho*, translated as "garlic wine" (see recipe on page 76). Virtually every meat-based Brazilian dish gets a preliminary baptism in garlic with this classic marinade and its distinctive smell that permeates city streets in Brazil during lunchtime and dinner. For homesick Brazilians, the fragrance of *vinha d'alho*—the combined aromas of garlic, wine, and bay leaf— serves as a Proustian madeleine. Garlic works well in the kitchen, but it works equally well from a health perspective. For several years now, cardiologists have touted garlic's power in reducing triglycerides and cholesterol in patients with heart disease and high blood pressure. Antibiotic, antifungal, and loaded with antioxidants, garlic trumps most other aromatics in benefits.

Guaraná [gwa-rah-NAH]

If you like sport or energy drinks, you may have come across *guaraná*. Native Amazonian *guaraná* berries can be dried and crushed to a powder or rendered into syrup, both of which enjoy popularity as potent energy-boosting supplements, and food and beverage additives. Brazilian *guaraná* enthusiasts rely on the berry for two functions: as a central nervous system stimulant, and as an aphrodisiac (although the latter is more legend than fact).

Many people enjoy *guaraná* for its delicate flavor. For most Brazilians, *guaraná* tastes best as a fizzy soft drink—and they consume it in quantities so large that *guaraná* soft drinks have outsold Coca-Cola in Brazil. The berry, when processed with a bit of cane sugar, tastes clean, fruity, and refreshing with a slight creamy nuttiness—similar to American cream soda. Cooks add *guaraná* syrups to desserts and smoothies, and fruit manufacturers infuse frozen fruit pulp with it to add a little kick.

Stimulant-packed *guaraná* contains caffeine and related chemicals, guaranine and theobromine, which are also found in chocolate. With *guaraná*, most people don't experience the kind of adverse reactions they have when drinking coffee. However, users of *guaraná* do report better stamina and energy.

There is a Brazilian Indian myth about the berry. According to the story, a Maués Indian couple gave birth to a boy who was as handsome and strong as he was kind. An evil spirit known as Jurupari grew jealous of the boy and, transformed into a serpent, bit and killed him. Tupã, the god of thunder, took pity on the couple and counseled them to plant the boy's eyes into the ground, from which a new plant would grow, bearing delicious fruits. So grew the *guaraná* plant, each of its small berries bearing an exact re-semblance to a human eye.

Guava, Papaya, and Pineapple, a.k.a. *Goiaba* [goy-AH-bah], *Mamão* [mah-MAOH], and *Abacaxi* [a-bah-kah-SHEE] or *Ananas* [ah-nah-NAHSS]

These fruits represent three of the most popular native fruits of Brazil. Widely eaten raw for breakfast, snacks, and dessert, or consumed in the forms of juices, ice creams, and jellies, these three fruits are as nutritious as they are delicious. Both pineapple and papaya are especially useful in promoting digestion because they contain enzymes that break down protein. The proteolytic actions of papain in papayas and bromelain in pineapples help to sooth gastrointestinal upsets, and both fruits demonstrate anti-inflammatory properties. The guava also has anti-inflammatory properties thanks to its high concentration of vitamin C. Due to Brazil's tropical climate, guava is often eaten as a delectable preserved paste, known as a *goiabada*. Brazil produces such an abundance of ripe fruit that preservation for long-term storage is essential; Brazilian supermarket aisles groan under the weight of multiple brands of guava pastes and banana preserves (known as *bananadas*). The rich *goiabada*, made from nothing more than fruit, water, and cane sugar, pairs well with cream cheese. Known as Romeo and Juliet (see recipe on page 102) this marriage of sweet and creamy flavors is a popular dessert or snack not only in Brazilian homes and restaurants, but also in many Central and South American countries as well as Portugal and Spain (which often substitutes quince for guava to make the resulting paste, *membrillo*).

Kale, a.k.a. *Couve* [KOH-vee] or Black Cabbage

When raw, the slightly bitter, mustardy kale can be somewhat of an acquired taste. But when cooked with a bit of olive oil, spicy pork sausage, and onion as Brazilians do, the kale yields a buttery sweetness that can become addictive. Kale's intense flavor and color star in such classically Portuguese and Brazilian dishes as Caldo Verde (see recipe on page 109) and Kale, Minas Style (see recipe on page 146). Of the four most com-monly used dark, leafy greens in Brazil (which also include watercress, spinach, and arugula), kale supercedes the others dramatically as the most robust in nutritional ben-efits. A source of iron, calcium, and vitamins B, C, and K, kale also contains carotenoid antioxidants in levels reputed to be among the highest found in any vegetable. As a member of the cancer-fighting cabbage family, kale contains a compound known as sul-foraphane (the source of kale's bitter, mustardy whiff), which in clinical studies has re-tarded breast cancer cell growth. Its high concentrations of vitamin A, lutein, and zeaxanthin may also aid in slowing such deteriorative vision problems as cataracts and macular degeneration. Kale's concentrations of vitamin K, a significant bone booster, can be very useful for menopausal women at risk for osteoporosis, since many American diets tend to be too low in amounts of the vitamin. A true superfood, kale's myriad health benefits provide many good reasons for incorporating the vegetable into the weekly menu—just as millions of Brazilians do.

Lime, a.k.a. *Limão, Lima Acida*

Brazil is one of the world's largest producers of limes, which is not surprising considering how integral limes and their juice are to the cuisine. Sadly, the limes most Brazilians consume daily are not easily available in the United States. In America, the typical commercially sold lime contains high levels of citric acid, whereas the common Brazilian lime has only very small amounts. In general, Brazilian limes are sweeter and fruitier, American limes are more tart and astringent. That should not stop you from cooking Brazilian dishes! Some reasonable substitutes can be found. I try to use Tahiti or Key limes, and add two drops of honey to every whole lime's juice. Regardless of the flavor, both kinds of limes provide important health benefits. Limonoids, the active compounds of the lime, appear to have potent cancer-fighting properties; limonoids also remain in the body for a far longer period on average than other tumor-battling phytosterols and phenols, such as those found in green tea. Like all citrus fruits, limes contain high concentrations of vitamin C—a powerful antioxidant and immune system booster.

Malagueta Peppers, a.k.a. *Pimenta*

Native to Brazil, the malagueta pepper plant grows wild in the Amazon river basin where it most likely originated. These low shrubs, bearing small, waxy, conical peppers, also grow on terraces, porches, and in sunny kitchens all over Brazil due to their hardiness and high fruit yield. The malagueta's closest relative is the Tabasco pepper, which offers similarities in flavor, heat, and appearance. Malaguetas can be found preserved whole in vinegar. When using these preserved peppers as a condiment, Brazilians rarely consume the pepper itself; rather, they add the pepper-infused vinegar to the food in small, careful drops. Malaguetas, like all fiery capsicums, have thermogenic (heat-producing) properties. The heat and sweating provoked by pepper consumption requires significant energy, so the body burns more calories. Capsaicin, the active substance that gives peppers their heat, is an anti-inflammatory that has been used for reducing arthritis pain and congestion. A rich source of vitamins A and C, peppers help to shore up the immune system and fight infection.

Manioc, a.k.a. *Mandioca* [man-jee-AW-kah], *Aipim* [eye-PEEM], *Macaxeira* [mah-kah-SHEH-rah], and *Farinha* [fah-REE-nyuh], or Yucca, Cassava, Tapioca

A starchy root native to South America, manioc was the primary foodstuff of Brazil's indigenous Amerindian population. Once colonizers arrived on Brazilian shores, they quickly added the myriad incarnations of manioc to their cuisine, thus deepening the cultural mélange of Brazilian gastronomy. Lethally toxic when raw, the manioc must first be boiled before its use (the cooking water, loaded with cyanide from the manioc's cyanogenic compounds, was often used by Indians as poison for hunting and fishing). Once boiled, it can be processed into such common products as tapioca for puddings, cakes, and stews; manioc chunks for making fries and mash (it's a good substitute for potatoes); and, most important, a flour that serves as the basis of biscuits, cakes, stews, and one of Brazil's most common dishes, *farofa*—which involves frying the manioc flour with eggs, bacon, and onion. Because manioc is a low-nutrition starch (and not so easy to find outside of Brazil), I've pointedly left out recipes for the fattening *farofa*, even though most Brazilians eat it once a day. However, if you wish to make it, simply pan-fry some chopped bacon and onion in a skillet until golden; add a cup of manioc flour and a little olive oil, stir it until completely incorporated; then crack one egg into the mixture and stir rapidly, until the egg cooks. Serve with rice.

Mate [MAH-chee], a.k.a. *Erva Mate* or *Matte,* or Yerba Maté

In the land of good coffee, excellent coffee substitutes abound. One of them is maté, a type of holly bush native to southern Brazil. When ground and steeped in boiling water, maté leaves produce an intensely flavored tea that energizes and calms. It also serves as an excellent substitute for people attempting to wean themselves off coffee or cola soft drinks. Smoky, oaky black tea flavors mix with a distinct hint of tobacco to create a drink that works well without sugar or milk, but tastes even better mixed with lime and a bit of sugar. The latter constitutes one of Brazil's most popular beverages, and commercial maté preparations with such additions as lime, *guaraná,* and other fruit flavors, crowd out carbonated soft drinks in most shops' cold drink cabinets. These drinks tout maté's potent antioxidant and mineral content (maté is rich in potassium, magnesium, and manganese), thereby reinforcing a centuries-old appreciation for maté as a healthy, revitalizing tonic.

Like coffee, maté contains alkaloids, chemical relatives to caffeine. However, like *guaraná,* maté's particular caffeine composition (xanthine alkaloids, also known as mateine) does not affect drinkers in the same way as that of coffee. Users experience similar levels of alertness and concentration, but without the jitters and palpitations. In fact, maté appears to relax smooth muscle tissue and stimulate the heart, rather than go right to the central nervous system. This paradoxical sedative-stimulant effect parallels maté's potential use as a calming antidepressant: In 2005, a trio of inventors filed a United States patent citing research into maté's efficacy in inhibiting monoamine oxidase activity in the brain—a key function also performed by pharmaceutical antidepressants.

Parsley, a.k.a. *Salsa*

Brazilians blend curly-leaf parsley with coriander and onion to make *cheiro verde*, a notably fragrant element in the country's cuisine. Beyond its flavoring uses, parsley packs important nutritional value. It might surprise you to know that parsley provides more vitamin C than oranges—more than twice as much, in fact. And while everyone praises spinach for its abundance of iron, parsley actually offers double the value. Like so many Brazilian ingredients, parsley is loaded with antioxidants, especially carotenoids, as well as such minerals as copper and manganese. But given the preponderance of such aromatics as garlic and onion in Brazilian cuisine, where parsley's star really shines is as nature's breath freshener! After a meal of *moqueca* (see recipe on page 130) or *frango à passarinho* (see recipe on page 141), be sure to grab a fresh sprig and chew away.

Salt Cod, a.k.a. *Bacalhau* [bah-kah-LYOW]

For the Portuguese, salting and drying their catches of "the beef of the sea" served as the only method by which cod could withstand long voyages to their far-flung imperial outposts. Once salt cod arrived on the shores of Brazil, it became a component of the diet. The locals prized the distinctive meatiness of this North Atlantic fish, a welcome addition to their already formidable stocks of South American river fish. Salt cod's rough, grayish hunks of stinky, hardened protein can offend sensitive souls with ginger constitutions, but they transform radically when prepared. Once the cod has been soaked for a day to remove the salt—this can be done in water, but I prefer milk—the cod swells to twice its size, virtually all traces of fishy odor gone. After soaking, salt cod flesh turns creamy, supple, and flaky, and it can then be poached, roasted, mashed, or fried. Best of all, for busy people on the go, *bacalhau* offers a great alternative to buying fresh fish on a regular basis—salt cod can be kept sealed in a cool, dry place for years without spoiling. A little goes a long way, thanks to its expansion when soaked, so you also can buy smaller amounts to make large meals. Unfortunately, due to overfishing, North Atlantic cod stocks have almost totally collapsed, thereby making Atlantic salt cod not much of an eco-friendly staple. Use Pacific cod (also known as scrod) or salted pollock instead, which can now be found in salted form, and use it as an occasional treat, no more than two to three times a month.

Palm Hearts, a.k.a. *Palmito* or Peach Palm

The tender inner flesh of the native Brazilian palm tree stem yields the delicious palm heart, a nutty, tangy vegetable that can be prepared in various ways. Many salads and soups feature the palm heart, its crunchy-creamy texture providing a counterpoint to the other ingredients. But I think it tastes best inside pies, either on its own or accompanying shrimp or chicken (see recipes on page 137). Treat it like a multipurpose substitute for asparagus, bamboo shoots, cucumber, and more. Rich in iron, vitamin A, folates, vitamin C, potassium, and phosphorus, the palm heart provides a fair amount of nutrition. Once harvested from *açaí* and other Brazilian native palms to the point of ecological disruption, commercial harvest of Brazilian palm hearts concentrates now on the pupunha palm, thanks to its rapid, sustainable growth and high yield. American stores typically stock the palm heart in cans, whereas in Brazil, shoppers buy it in transparent glass jars. Both preserve the delicate flavor of the vegetable and its characteristic texture.

Pumpkin, a.k.a. *Abobora* [ah-BAW-boh-rah]

I've always found it strange that despite the American pumpkin's native roots, most people in the United States only consume it during the holidays. In Brazil, cooks revere the versatile pumpkin for its use in savories and desserts all year round. It appears in luxuriously sweet candies, marmalades, puddings, and cakes, usually alongside coconut; in unsweetened form, the pumpkin's flesh may be cooked down in stews, boiled and mashed, or simply put aside so that the squash itself can be stuffed with other ingredients. The pumpkin's flesh and oil impart uses beyond gustatory; sometimes soothing pumpkin poultices are made to treat parasitic infections. Pumpkin products have been used for centuries in Brazil to treat tapeworm and other invaders. The nutritionally rich seeds currently attract the most attention for their potent efficacy in treating prostate hyperplasia (enlarged prostate). Because the disorder occurs as a result of a chemical malfunction that also leads to premature hair loss, pumpkin seeds have demonstrated worth in slowing balding, too.

Watercress, a.k.a. *Agrião* [ah-gree-YUNH]

A close relative to kale, watercress bears a similar mustardy, sulphurous base note in its flavor. Brazilians use the distinctively peppery taste of watercress for more than salad leaves; watercress appears as a flavoring in stews, sauces, and soups. Rich in vitamins A and C, as well as antioxidants and such minerals as calcium, iodine, and iron, watercress acts as a stimulant. Bikini-conscious Brazilians also rely on watercress for its diuretic properties.

Inside the Melting Pot

People like to use the metaphor of a melting pot when describing areas in which people of different races and cultures come together. Historians, statisticians, and poets most frequently invoke the name of New York City as the quintessential melting pot, given its history as the busiest port of global immigration at the turn of the twentieth century. While it's true that New York is indeed a place where every possible language, religion, creed, and cuisine might be found among its population, its status as a true melting pot pales in comparison to that of Brazil's.

Brazil's gene pool contains a global mix of Amerindian, European, African, Middle Eastern, and Asian DNA. Thanks to successive waves of colonization and immigration, coupled with a tropical climate and a nationally libertine disposition that courts a lot of nooky, a typical Brazilian could range in shade from Nordic blond and blue-eyed to amaretto-skinned and green-eyed, coffee-colored and black-eyed, even black-skinned and red-haired.

So it is with Brazilian cuisine. The building blocks of Brazilian cuisine reflect the myriad influences of its people and cultures, fused together to make an amalgam that exhibits traces of each constituent element, but which stands on its own as a unique, cohesive gastronomic whole. Consider the most prominent sources of ethnic diversity that fuel the eating habits of this giant, five-hundred-year-old nation:

Amerindian. The indigenous people of Brazil, representing approximately two thousand different tribes at the time of Brazil's discovery by the Portuguese in 1500, were—and a much diminished population continues to be—seminomadic hunters and gatherers. Subsisting on the plentiful supplies of fish, animals, fruit, nuts, and seeds of the vast Brazilian interior, they focused much of their agricultural cultivation around the native manioc or cassava root. The starchy tuber was used for making flour and alcohol then and, to this day, remains a primary staple in Brazilian cuisine. Tapioca, manioc flour, and manioc root are all important carbohydrate elements of the daily Brazilian diet.

Portuguese. The Portuguese were the first of many Western Europeans, especially the French, Dutch, and Spanish, to arrive on Brazilian shores. Their culinary legacy stamped one of the strongest influences on the cuisine, donating classic dishes made with salt cod, the pork sausage known as *chouriço*, and kale. The Portuguese tradition of using wine or vinegar to marinate and cook still exists in the use of *vinha d'alho* (Garlic Wine Marinade—see recipe on page 76). The Portuguese also brought with them their legendary affinity for supersweet desserts made with eggs and sugar. When they added local Brazilian coconut to their traditional egg custards, such classically Brazilian desserts like *quimdim* were born.

African. Taken predominantly from western Africa, with many Brazilian slaves coming from the Yoruba and Bantu people, Africans left an important and vital imprint on both Brazilian cultural history and its cuisine. They brought with them such staples as the African *dendê* palm for oil; a taste for cooking with such native African ingredients as okra, peanuts, and black-eyed peas; and a strong sense of how to make the best and most delicious uses of offal. Brought to the northeastern coastal town of Bahia, the center of sugar production and thus the main port of entry for the Brazilian slave trade (slaves were brought in fewer numbers to the ports of Recife and Rio de Janeiro), Africans made their Afro-Brazilian hybrid cuisine one of the country's most distinct culinary branches. But Africans played an even bigger role in shaping Brazilian food as we know it today. Slaves brought to the kitchens to cook for their Portuguese, French, or Dutch masters were responsible for fusing their owners' national dishes and taste preferences with whatever local ingredients were at hand—making the Africans the real creative forces that shaped much of what we recognize as Brazilian food today. For example, the word *quimdim*, the name of the glossy and sweet egg-and-coconut pie cited in the Portuguese section above, comes from the Bantu dialect and means "having the demeanor of a teenage girl."

Italian. Italian immigrants made their way to Brazil in large numbers from the 1880s to around 1930. Indeed, over 25 million Brazilians are of Italian heritage, and they constitute the fourth most significant Brazilian ethnic heritage after Amerindians, Portuguese, and Africans. Italians settled mainly in the south and southeastern regions of Brazil, primarily to work on coffee plantations. Among the lasting gastronomic imprints they've made on Brazilian cuisine are the use of and popularity of pizza, polenta, lasagne, and pasta—in addition to the cultural legacies left in the form of language. Even now, Brazilians say *tchau* (*ciao*) when they bid you farewell.

Japanese. In 1908, the *Kasato Maru* sailed from Kobe, Japan, to Santos, Brazil, with 791 Japanese emigrants hoping to find work in the coffee plantations of southern Brazil near São Paulo. Over time, more immigrants arrived, making the current millions of Japanese Brazilians living in Brazil the largest group of people of Japanese descent outside of Japan. Today, around 300,000 Japanese Brazilians live in Japan (contrast that with the estimated 800,000 Japanese in the United States). Japanese Brazilians serve an important role in the agricultural business of Brazil, and they exert a strong influence on the cultural and industrial forces that link the two nations. Elements of Japanese cuisine are very popular aspects of Brazilian gastronomy. For example, Brazilian barbecue houses uniformly serve sushi, sashimi, and Japanese vegetables and salads as part of their buffet offerings. Most big urban supermarkets sell packets of dashi and miso (*misso* in Portuguese) required to prepare miso soup, along with *furikake* (the mix of seaweed, spices, dried fish and shrimp, and sesame seeds used to season boiled rice), nori, and other basic ingredients.

Middle Eastern. Immigrants from Syria, Lebanon, and Palestine started arriving in Brazil during the latter half of the nineteenth century to work on farms and plantations like so many of the other ethnic groups that came seeking opportunity. They brought with them a vibrant cuisine featuring baked goods, pastries, meat dishes, and salads that have become part of Brazil's culinary vernacular. Walk into any snack shop, juice bar, or bakery in the south or southeastern regions and you'll find *esfihas*, doughy triangles of puffy bread stuffed with meat and cheese. Chances are you'll also find *quibe* (see recipe on page 98)—kibbe, a type of fried or roasted meatball—right next to the *esfihas*. The passion for Middle Eastern flavors has integrated so well in Brazil that Habib's, a restaurant franchise serving *esfihas*, *quibe*, hummus, and more, has emerged as one of Brazil's most popular fast-food options.

Northern European. Settlers from Germany, Switzerland, Finland, and elsewhere made their distinctive marks on Brazil and its culture (and not just in the form of supermodel Gisele Bündchen). In 1827, the first settlers arrived from Germany settling in Rio Grande do Sul in the south. Over time, more Northern European immigrants arrived and built towns that closely resembled those they left behind in Europe. Visitors who travel to such Brazilian destinations as Blumenau and Guarei in the south and mountain towns such as Novo Friburgo and Petropolis farther north in Rio de Janeiro state can see wooden chalets and buildings that bear the characteristic Saxon and Swiss architectural styles, and German is still spoken in many of these areas. Each year, Blumenau hosts an enormous Oktoberfest. Beer, fondue, potato salad, dumplings, and spice cakes are popular food items that have been absorbed into Brazil's gastronomic culture.

I want to emphasize that the BBBP is a lifestyle book, a road map for improving your existence, as opposed to a diet book. You won't find calorie counts beside the recipes. The minute eating becomes a chore, like homework, the incentive to stick with a program disappears. I want readers to focus on the ingredients of their food and how it smells and tastes, restoring a sensual pleasure and joy to eating. The goal of the BBBP is to reeducate readers on how to eat wholesome, delicious food in reasonable-size portions, and how to balance food intake with movement so that weight fluctuation stabilizes, thereby eliminating constant calculation.

As frames of reference, Brazil and Brazilian cuisine serve as ideal models for this reeducation. The Brazilian diet contains the ultimate superfood ingredients—plentiful in fruit and vegetables, legumes, fish and lean meats. The world's biggest agricultural powerhouse, Brazil grows some of the most nutritious and delicious plants on Earth. Many of these are native and exclusive to Brazil, such as *açaí*, cashews and Brazil nuts, maté tea, *guaraná*, and more. The basic staples that constitute the cuisine are almost uniformly the food chain's richest sources of vitamins and antioxidants. Brazilian food is not only highly nutritious, it also underscores a social eating culture that places a high value on dining seated at a table with family and friends.

In America, where advertising and car dependency have conspired to turn fast food into a legitimate daily dining option, eating has been stripped of nutrition, taste, and conviviality. In their stead lie giant, double-stuffed portions with extra cheese, "man food," and oil drum–size tubs of sugary soft drinks or coffee, all gulped down by often solitary drivers behind the wheel of a car. No wonder the country's obesity problem is out of control.

Many claim convenience as the primary reason behind their willingness to consume massive quantities of fatty foods, though corporate and political interests also lie subliminally at the heart of the push to get customers to eat this way. But there's nothing convenient about the cancer that's growing at the heart of American society: The American population is fatter, at greater risk of heart disease and musculoskeletal problems, and consequently saddling itself with the ever-increasing burden of stratospheric health-care costs to manage the results of its obsession with junk food. The food choices you make not only have a direct effect on you, but also on everyone else around you—whether they shorten and directly affect your quality of life and that of those you love, or drive up insurance costs for your fellow citizens.

We now live in an age of great uncertainty, and our unwillingness to confront the effects of our individual choices is coming back to haunt us: Our perverse relationship with food and sloth has made type 2 diabetes the most serious epidemic confronting the nation; our mania for gigantic, gas-guzzling cars and deforestation have warmed the earth to the point of provoking more frequent killer droughts, storms, and floods; our disinterest in conservation has turned beautiful countryside into ugly shopping malls or areas of fossil fuel extraction and refinement to satisfy an insatiable petro-lust; our reflexive inability to view ourselves as others see us and to honestly address this gap has spurred aggression and hatred worldwide.

The time has come for taking the first step toward global change, no matter how small. With the BBBP, I suggest a path focused on taking responsibility for your own body, as well as for the impact your food and exercise choices have on others. Follow it to the best of your ability, and you'll see improvement in your weight and muscle tone. You'll feel lighter and happier. You'll improve your chances of living a longer life of better quality. Your use of certain products will make a very small but important contribution to the conservation of plant life critical to the existence of the Amazon. Think of it as your investment in the future—yours and the world's.

Sucos and Other Food Tidbits

Food, a deeply primal love and respect for it and the sensual pleasures it brings, lies at the instinctive heart of Brazilian culture—much as it does in places like France, Italy, Spain, and Japan. In Brazil, the food experience comes in a dazzling array of forms.

Sophisticated restaurants in São Paulo and Rio vie with those in New York or Paris for innovation in preparation and chic crowds of diners; weekly markets in every city and town explode with color, fragrance, and hustle—especially in the North where copious piles of fruit and fish from the Amazon astonish outsiders with their memorable exoticism; street food vendors trundle carts bearing delicious homemade savories and desserts, the apotheosis of which are the mobile kitchens of the distinctively white-robed cheeky and chatty women of Bahia who sell their ambrosial Afro-Brazilian treats; beach-side food vendors are in a class by themselves, offering everything from cold *caipirinhas* to barbecued shrimp with lime sauce to barbecued cheese—and they carry their smoking mini-barbecues with them; *botequims,* the lively open-air pubs that serve the country's famous, tapas-like *salgadinhos* ("little salty things") with the Brazilian beer known as *chopp* (served *estupidamente gelada,* or "stupidly cold"), draw packs of partiers postwork until dawn.

Without a doubt, my favorite expression of Brazilian food mania is the corner juice bar, or *casa de sucos* ("house of juices"). Much like Italian espresso bars, these fabulous destinations usually have no chairs or tables, or doors. They are designed to serve people who breeze in off the streets for a quick snack to be eaten or drunk standing up. After purchasing a ticket, customers belly up to the counter, usually decorated with an eye-popping architectural display of fresh fruits, and place an order for anything from a frosty glass of freshly pulped fruit, to an espresso and a cheese roll or sandwich, to more substantial fare like set meals on a plate (*prato feito*) consisting of grilled meat, rice, beans, french fries, salad, and more.

Whenever I return to Brazil, my morning ritual consists of a walk or run along the beach, followed by a post-workout breakfast of an *açaí* smoothie known as an Automatic Pilot at one of my favorite juice bars in Rio, Big Nectar. As delightful as the drink is, part of the pleasure in drinking it is watching life unfold at the juice bar. Workers grab a quick *cafezinho* and croissant before heading to their offices; surfers back from the early dawn action on the breaks at Rio's Arpoador hunch over their *açaí* bowls, their boards leaning against the counter; deliverymen haul aromatic crates of mangoes, pineapples, limes, and more over the counter to the juicers to be pulped; tourists gaze up at the impenetrable juice menu boards studded with Amazonian fruit names they can't recognize or pronounce; the baristas behind the counter busily prepare drinks, sandwiches, pizzas, and the delicate fried savory pockets known as *pasteis,* all while bantering with and good-naturedly ribbing the customers.

Corner juice bars are like pubs in the United Kingdom. Each one has its distinctive crowd of regulars. For example, my other favorite juice bar in Rio, BiBi Sucos, is world famous for being the hangout of choice for professional surfers and Brazilian jiu-jitsu stars, whose signed head shots grace the walls underneath the two suspended flat screen televisions showing surf, jiu-jitsu, and judo competitions.

The ritual of popping in at the juice bar for a healthy (and occasionally unhealthy) snack underscores a few habits Brazilians have about food. They might have a coffee at a juice bar, but this simple act stands in diametric opposition to the way in which Americans, for example, drink coffee. Whereas a stop at an American Starbucks might involve loafing on a sofa with an enormous portion of sugary, milky coffee, Brazilians—true coffee lovers—take a quick, small shot of espresso as a booster, and then they're off again.

The BBBP doesn't necessarily advocate the habit of coffee-drinking; if you need the energy boost from caffeine, try an Automatic Pilot (see recipe on page 65) or a glass of maté instead. By all means, if you want to occasionally savor a good coffee, Brazilian style, one every now and then won't hurt. But regular, excessive coffee drinking dehydrates the system and can make people too jittery. Worse, coffee consumption that takes the form of cutesy-named, milky dessert drinks load your body with sugar and fat on top of the caffeine.

Speaking of milky coffee drinks, Brazilians aren't in the habit of drinking much milk, either. Dairy products are used more for cooking, rather than drinking, and, even then, milk rarely makes an appearance. However, cheese, cream, and condensed milk play a big role in the cuisine, serving as a base for sauces and desserts. For Americans and Europeans used to seeing cartons of fresh milk front and center in supermarkets, it's a bit of a shock to see that in Brazil, many dairy products tend to come out of cans—a necessity that developed as a result of the climate and limited refrigeration resources.

The BBBP tries to harness a lot of very good Brazilian food habits, while also discarding a few less beneficial ones. Among the habits you'd be well advised to steer clear from is the Brazilian scheduling of dinner. As in many European and South American countries, the last meal of the day might be eaten as late as ten or eleven in the evening—and you can bet it will be a big one, too. For people who lead a sedentary lifestyle, this is the quickest way to gain weight. While following the BBBP, do not eat for at least three hours before bedtime. Sometimes this is unavoidable, so if you are having a late meal, keep it light and be sure to do a BBBP Full-Hour Workout the following day.

Another alteration of Brazilian eating habits concerns the use of white rice. I admit I prefer the taste of white rice over brown, but brown rice is a good way of getting whole grains into your diet. So when cooking, try whenever you can to substitute good brown rice for white. If you dislike regular brown rice, try using a brown rice like Texmati, a whole-grain brown rice that looks, cooks, and tastes more like white rice. Be sure to eat only whole-grain bread and pasta.

As for good Brazilian habits, one is the regular daily use of legumes. People who know little of Brazilian cuisine expect the use of black beans, but are less familiar with the popularity of such legumes as chickpeas, lentils, black-eyed peas, and peanuts. All of these appear frequently on the Brazilian menu, in various preparations. Their versatility is matched only by their benefits. More important, beans are cheap, and provide an excellent source of nutrition when you need to be frugal with your culinary budget. A complex carbohydrate, beans keep you fuller longer, and they provide stores of energy rapidly depleted by stressful lifestyles. They can be used in soups, salads, purees, fritters, and much more. The BBBP offers several ways of eating them that should please even the fussiest of eaters. As an occasional treat, I urge you to try *acarajé* (see recipe on page 100), the Bahian fritter made from black-eyed peas. Once tasted, it's never forgotten.

One final positive Brazilian habit to develop (and one that gives you a good excuse to make *acarajé*) is to hone your entertaining skills. Brazilians love to regularly host people for dinner, a barbecue, or a coffee or tea. To the Brazilian mind, preparing food for others is a demonstration of affection and generosity—as well as a way of showcasing deft skills with layered flavors. Some Brazilian recipes can only be effectively prepared for eating with a group—take *feijoada* (see recipe on page 123) as an example. Adopting the Brazilian social approach to dining can be a great way for you to reconnect with family and friends. Brazilians are extremely family-oriented culturally—a fact that can be observed on weekends at any good restaurant. Tables are overwhelmingly for four or more people, populated by several generations of a family out for their regular weekly lunch or dinner get-together.

Eating and Weight

It's possible to entertain and enjoy food and still lose weight. Let's face it, the mathematics of weight control is pretty simple. You must take in fewer calories than you burn. The average man at rest burns anywhere from 2,200 to 2,900 calories per day. The total daily energy expenditure for an average women at rest is anywhere from 1,700 to 2,100. Both these figures are based on sedentary Americans. A lot of range exists in these figures, depending on whether you are overweight and inactive (you'll burn fewer calories) to very lean and athletic (you'll burn far more). To lose weight, you need to take in approximately 400–500 calories less than your total daily energy expenditure each day—that's the equivalent of going without that jump-starting frappaccino, or morning bagel and afternoon candy bar.

Because losing a pound of fat requires burning approximately 3,500 calories, you'll need to consume 500 calories less than your total daily energy expenditure per day for one week, to drop one pound. That's assuming you do no exercise at all. A pound a week might seem inconsequential, but if you raised your activity level—even if it's for ten minutes—by doing some moderate exercise each day while keeping your caloric intake stable or decreasing it within reason, your rate of weight loss will go up accordingly. Eat less, exercise more, and off come the pounds. The BBBP is an ideal way to help you achieve those goals.

While I advocate a Brazilian cultural model to help you change your life, I am not suggesting Brazilians are perfect. Obesity rates are exploding there as they are in the United States, United Kingdom, France, China, and other countries. Brazil, thanks to an increase in fast-food joints and soft drink consumption as well as growing urbanization and economic stability that causes the rates of inactivity to rise, is facing a fatter future. As one of the largest sugar consumers in the world (on par with the United States), Brazil doesn't always make the best use of its own advantages, even when those advantages include production of and affinity for the staples of the world's best diet.

While the ingredients and recipes of this program are authentically Brazilian, I've altered the structure of Brazilian menu combinations in such a way as to maximize nutrition and avoid the pitfalls of fatty, sugary, and starchy excess common to the country. For example, a typical Brazilian meal might include a lean piece of grilled turkey with a salad and black beans, but it will also certainly come with white rice, fried manioc flour, and maybe even some fried potatoes. And Brazilians have an incomparable sweet tooth, luxuriating in delicious desserts that feature eggs and sugar in the most sinful ways.

While I don't eliminate any item in particular (except for maybe fried manioc flour, although you'll find a brief recipe for it on page 25), I do modify the food groupings to lessen the ratio of starch to protein. I encourage you to use whole-grain versions of certain starches like brown rice for white, and whole-wheat bread or wraps instead of white bread and rolls. Reduced-fat dairy may replace full fat. Sweeteners may replace sugar (try to stick with natural sweeteners like stevia or agave syrup, if possible, but Splenda also does the trick). Most important, be careful about your serving sizes. Portion sizes must be kept in control—in general, individual portions of meat or fish should be about the size of a fist and no thicker than two inches. A "handful" portion means exactly that and no more. Soup servings are one cup and no more. But I make all of these recommendations with the caveat that, in some cases, you may and should allow yourself the occasional indulgence. Life without it is poor and joyless. In short, the BBBP's food is recognizably Brazilian, but I've used the building blocks of dishes to create a nutritional structure lighter and more flexible than the one used by many Brazilians.

The BBBP can help families change their habits together by providing complete instructions on how to construct savory, nutritious meals with one another. It encourages dining and exercising as group activities. It urges you to have fun. And it dictates flexibility: Get through it the best you can. If you can't manage all of it, improvise. And keep smiling.

PEDRO MÜLLER

Professional surfer and director of the Pedro Müller Starpoint Surf School in Rio de Janeiro. As national surf champion in 1988 and 1992, Müller distinguished himself even further by being one of the oldest winners of this young-person's sport (he won the national title at thirty-eight). As the director of ABRASP (Brazilian Professional Surf Association), Müller continues to oversee some of the surf world's biggest competitions.

I've been lucky to establish a really good equilibrium between the activities and people in my life. Living a healthy life, getting up and going to bed early, eating good nutritious food, allows me to be at peace.

I surf practically every day, with the exception of Monday, which is my day of rest when I try not to do any activities in the ocean. I also work out from Monday through Friday. I tend to alternate between lifting weights and doing yoga. I insist on my students working out and stretching before they go into the water and afterward, so at the school I have a yoga teacher who helps lead the exercise sessions on the beach.

I am very serious about what I eat because of what I do. In the morning, I'll have some orange juice and granola. I love oatmeal, yogurt, whole wheat breads, and especially soy protein—I mix it with banana and papaya, the fruits I eat the most. I also eat a lot of açaí, which I love, mixed with a bit of banana. Lunch is usually my biggest meal—I always eat rice, beans, fish, and salad. I also eat good red meat because I'm a skinny guy and I burn a lot of calories every day. If I left red meat out, I'd be skin and bones. So I eat everything. If I'm competing, I eat pasta for carbohydrates. On the weekends, when I'm relaxing with my family, I'll indulge a bit, have a few beers. My family and I also love Japanese food and eat a lot of it. And yes, I do eat desserts, especially anything with bananas, or cakes made with chocolate or carrot.

I think that in general Brazilians are people who live with great intensity, despite a lot of social problems that divide the very wealthy and the very poor. Brazilians speak loudly, love to have fun, love to eat and socialize. Compared to Europeans or Americans, we're a noisy bunch! But we love being surrounded by our friends and family the most. Having the weekend lunch with your extended family is a tradition here, which I think is really cool. It's a worthy value.

The Amazon's Wealth on Your Table

In Brazil's Amazon region, the impressive landscapes of states like Pará and Amazonas feature views of lush riverside *açaí* palm groves, crowded with majestic, seventy-foot-tall trees heavy with six-foot-long fruit-bearing spathes. The palm, known as an *açaízeiro* in Portuguese, and its blue-black fruit are indigenous to Brazil. An old saying in Portuguese goes, "He who went to Pará, stopped. He who tasted *açaí*, stayed."

The magnificent *açaí* is just one reason why people marvel at the Amazon. Seductively exotic, this primeval forest is so vast (even in spite of its rapid destruction) and so bountiful that it contains an estimated 30 percent of the world's total number of animal species and over forty thousand identified plants—and new species are discovered every year. Indeed, the size, complexity, and partial inaccessibility of the Amazon preserve its unknowable mystique.

The Amazon's mind-boggling yield of useful plants ranges from species of shrubs, to vines, to massive evergreen trees whose canopies house the birds and animals that help keep the vegetation multiplying. But let's first take a look at one of the most functional groups of Amazon plants: palms.

The palm botanical family, known as Arecaceae, supplies us with some of our most prized food products: coconuts, palm oil, hearts of palm, and more. The BBBP bases its recipes on all of these delicious and nutritious products, but one palm product stands above the rest and that is *açaí*.

For Amazon dwellers, the *açaí* is suitable for every conceivable use. Its fronds, wood, and spathes serve as sturdy and insect-repelling construction material for housing, bridges, river pontoons, bags and baskets, household brooms, even hats. But it's the fruit that can have the most impact on your life.

Açaí provides one of nature's most valuable nutrition sources wrapped in a tiny, marble-size package. It's rich in such minerals as calcium, phosphorus, potassium, and iron, and in vitamins A, B_1, B_2, B_3, C, and E. The unctuous pulp is high in protein and loaded with omega-6 and omega-9 fatty acids, as well as small amounts of the precious omega-3 fatty acids that most diets sorely lack. Much of the excitement around *açaí* revolves around the fruit's anthocyanins—the compounds that give the berry its distinctive blue-black color and its significantly high levels of antioxidants.

Commercial packagers of *açaí* tout levels of antioxidants almost double that of blueberries and more than ten times that of red wine. Antioxidants are measured in a unit known as an ORAC (oxygen radical absorption capacity). While no United States Department of Agriculture (USDA) mandates on total daily antioxidant consumption levels currently exist, research conducted by scientists at the Jean Mayer USDA Human Nutrition Center on Aging, at Tufts University in Boston, Massachusetts, suggest that the human body needs between 3,000 and 5,000 ORACs per day for significant antioxidant activity. A typical day's nutrition provides around 1,600 ORACs daily. But some commercial preparations of pure *açaí* pulp provide ORAC levels as high as 5,700.

Years of medicinal *açaí* use in the Amazon region anecdotally attest to the berry's power as a potent force in combating digestive and intestinal problems, as well as skin disorders. Other parts of the plant are used for healing, too, such as the palm heart (for stopping bleeding gums) and the *açaí* root (antiwormers). Very little clinical research on *açaí* exists, primarily because *açaí* is highly perishable. Within twenty-four hours of having been picked, the *açaí* berry oxidizes to the point at which most of its nutrients are rendered inactive. Widespread commercial *açaí* processing for export, which involves immediate pulping and freezing of the berry, has only been available for the last seven years, so official studies are few and far between. However, a recent study shows strong initial evidence supporting the anecdotal reports of *açaí*'s powerful effect on human tissue.

In January 2006, researchers at University of Florida's Institute of Food and Agricultural Sciences, in Gainesville, Florida, published their study of *açaí* on cultured human cancer cells. When leukemia cell cultures were exposed to *açaí*, the berry extract triggered a self-destruct response in 86 percent of the cells tested. While this in no way is evidence of *açaí* as a cure for cancer, it is a promising first step in isolating clinical information about how *açaí* benefits the body.

You don't need scientists to confirm one aspect of *açaí*'s goodness. The taste makes it a very popular and addictive treat. *Açaí* berries have a flavor similar to chocolate-covered cherries. Caffeine and theobromine, the active caffeine relative found in cacao, give the fruit an energy kick that makes *açaí* the food of choice among Brazil's athletes. The berry's consistency makes it ideal for puddings, ice creams, and other desserts, but most people eat the pulp as a frozen slush mixed with *guaraná*, granola, and other fruits like strawberries and bananas.

The BBBP strives to provide users with a meal plan that is as high as possible in antioxidants, vitamins, and minerals. To accomplish this, *açaí* is featured as a daily breakfast item, in the form of a shake called the Automatic Pilot (see recipe on page 65). Making an Automatic Pilot your daily breakfast ritual is the easiest way to start incorporating the BBBP into your life. Try it and see why *açaí* is fast becoming one of the most popular new fruits outside of Brazil.

Açaí is not the only nutritionally important Amazon product featured in the BBBP. As already discussed, nuts like cashews and Brazil nuts, the acerola cherry, coconuts, guava, papaya, and more feature in the recipes and menus to bring you both flavor and good nutrients. With the possible exception of acerola, these ingredients should be familiar to you. But these are only just a tiny fraction of the Amazon's staggering food bounty. In the following section, you'll find a very small sampling of Brazil's plentitude from the rainforest and beyond, most of which you will never see outside of Brazil (although some are now available through mail order; see Resources). Many of these unfamiliar and delicious fruits contain properties and nutrition almost as considerable as *açaí*. Scan through them to acquaint yourself with the incredible riches the world is lucky to have—and which we could lose if we don't take action now to preserve what remains of the Amazon. Half the fun is just rolling around the native Indian names of the fruits on your tongue, which is almost as delightful as sampling the fruits themselves.

A SHORT GUIDE TO BRAZILIAN FRUIT

Abiu [ah-BYOO], a.k.a. Eggfruit
FOOD USES: Smoothies, puddings, and ice creams—lime juice often used to balance out the *abiu*'s sweetness
MEDICINAL USES: Used in treating respiratory disorders
VITAMINS: High in vitamin C
MINERALS: Calcium, phosphorus

Araçá-Boi [ah-rah-SAH BOY]
FOOD USES: Fruit drinks, marmalades, fruit pastes, and ice cream
VITAMINS: Vitamins A, B_1, and C
MINERALS: Calcium, phosphorus

Biribá [bee-ree-BAH]
FOOD USES: Smoothies, ice creams, and wine
MEDICINAL USES: Stimulant and antiscorbutic (scurvy preventive)
VITAMINS: Extremely high in vitamin C. Contains vitamins B_1 and B_2, and traces of vitamin B_3
MINERALS: Calcium, phosphorus

Buriti [boo-ree-CHEE]
FOOD USES: Juices, puddings, oil, ice creams, and wine; mixed with manioc flour to make candies
MEDICINAL USES: Laxative and cure for diarrhea, treatment for vitamin A deficiency
VITAMINS: Vitamins A and C
MINERALS: Rich in oleic acids

Cacau [ka-KOW], a.k.a. Cacao
FOOD USES: Pulp used in juices, smoothies, sweets, puddings, ice creams; seeds or "beans" used in making butter, chocolate, and candies
MEDICINAL USES: Used as skin-softener, diuretic, stimulant, and aphrodisiac
VITAMINS: Vitamins B_1 and B_2
MINERALS: Rich in iron and magnesium; beans contain high concentrations of antioxidants, caffeine-like alkaloids, serotonin, tryptophan, and dopamine—all of which together produce the chocolate "high"

Cajá [ka-ZHAH] or *Taperebá* [tah-peh-reh-BAH], a.k.a. Hogplum
FOOD USES: Juices, compotes, jellies, syrups, and wine; used in cocktails
MEDICINAL USES: High water content makes it a thirst-reliever; diuretic and treatment for stomachaches
VITAMINS: High in vitamin C
MINERALS: High in calcium and potassium

Caju [ka-ZHOO], a.k.a. Cashew Apple
FOOD USES: The *caju* peduncle is used for juices, cakes, sweets, puddings, fruit pastes, jellies, ice creams, and liqueurs; the nut is used for flour, oil, butter, and candy
MEDICINAL USES: Antiseptic and diuretic; treatment for diarrhea, inflammation, and high blood pressure; soothes digestive upsets
VITAMINS: High in vitamins C and B_2
MINERALS: Iron and phosphorus; excellent source of pectin

Camu-Camu [ka-MOO ka-MOO]
FOOD USES: Juices and jellies, frozen desserts
MEDICINAL USES: Used to make Vitamin C pills
VITAMINS: High in vitamin C, as well as vitamins A, B_1, and B_2
MINERALS: High in potassium

Cupuaçu [koo-poo-ah-SOO]
FOOD USES: Juices, jellies, chocolates, puddings, and ice creams; seeds used to make butter and white chocolate
MEDICINAL USES: Treatment for abdominal pain; Amerindians use it to ease difficult childbirths
VITAMINS: Vitamins A, B_1, B_2, C, and E
MINERALS: High in calcium, iron, and magnesium

Fruta-do-Conde [froo-tah doo KAWN-djeh] or *Pinha* [PEEN-nyah], a.k.a. Sugar Apple, Custard Apple, Sweetsop
FOOD USES: Juices, smoothies, and ice creams
MEDICINAL USES: Appetite stimulant; seeds used to make insecticides
VITAMINS: Vitamins A, B_3, and C
MINERALS: Calcium and phosphorus

Gabiroba [gah-bee-RAW-buh]

FOOD USES: Juices, puddings, ice creams, and cocktails

MEDICINAL USES: Used to treat gastrointestinal disorders, diarrhea, and urinary tract infections

VITAMINS: Vitamin C

MINERALS: Source of pectin

Graviola [grah-vee-AW-lah], a.k.a. Soursop

FOOD USES: Juices, smoothies, puddings, ice creams, and cocktails

MEDICINAL USES: Used to treat inflammation and cancer

VITAMINS: Vitamins A, B_1, B_2, B_3, and C

MINERALS: High in calcium, phosphorus, and zinc

Jabuticaba [zhah-boo-chee-KAH-bah]

FOOD USES: Juices, puddings, ice creams, and cocktails

MEDICINAL USES: Appetite stimulant and energy booster; used to treat rheumatism and skin disorders

VITAMINS: Vitamins B_2 B_3, and C

MINERALS: Calcium, iron, and phosphorus

Jenipapo [zhen-ee-PAH-po]

FOOD USES: Juices, candies, jellies, and ice creams

MEDICINAL USES: Used to treat anemia, liver, and digestive problems

VITAMINS: Vitamin C

MINERALS: High in calcium, iron, and phosphorus

Maracujá [mah-rah-koo-ZHAH], a.k.a. Passion Fruit

FOOD USES: Juices, smoothies, puddings, cakes, jellies, cocktails, and ice creams

MEDICINAL USES: Relieves diarrhea; used as a sedative

VITAMINS: Vitamins A and C

MINERALS: High in iron, potassium, and zinc

Pitanga [pee-TUNH-guh], a.k.a. Brazil Cherry

FOOD USES: Juices, smoothies, puddings, jellies, cocktails, and wine

MEDICINAL USES: Used to treat beri-beri (disease caused by vitamin B_1 deficiency); leaves are fever-reducers

VITAMINS: Vitamins B_1 and C
MINERALS: High in zinc

Pupunha [poo-POON-nyuh]

FOOD USES: Juices, smoothies, cake flour, jellies, ice creams, oil, and wine; the stem of the tree is harvested for palm hearts
MEDICINAL USES: Relieves diarrhea
VITAMINS: Vitamins A, B_1, and C
MINERALS: High in calcium, iron, phosphorus, potassium, and zinc

Umbu [oom-BOO]

FOOD USES: Juices, sweets, fruit pastes, ice creams, vinegar, and wine
MEDICINAL USES: Thirst- and hunger-quencher
VITAMINS: Vitamins A and C
MINERALS: Calcium, iron, and phosphorus

Uxi [oo-SHEE]

FOOD USES: Fruit pastes, liqueurs, and ice creams; often mixed with manioc flour when eaten raw
MEDICINAL USES: Fever reducer
VITAMINS: Excellent source of vitamin E
MINERALS: Rich in fiber and phytoestrogens

Tools for the Kitchen

To follow the BBBP, a reasonable amount of food preparation needs to get done, but a few hours each week is sufficient to cover the bulk of the kitchen work.

I've compiled a list of the basic elements you'll need to outfit your kitchen properly for maximum efficiency in food preparation. Some, perhaps many, of these items may already be at your disposal. But take the time to look through the list to see where gaps remain and where redundancies may exist. Some of the equipment cited is, in fact, redundant to the others, but some redundant tools work better in certain circumstances. For example, a food processor and an onion dicer do the same thing, but if you're looking to dice one onion for lunch, a quick motion of a dicer will get the job done in a second. It's not worth it to haul out the food processor, switch it on, and clean it afterward for just one onion. Food processors are a better option when you need to cut ten onions rather than one. Remember that some tools with similar capabilities suit different needs.

The list is set up in two categories: Must-Haves and a Wish List. The items in the Wish List are not imperative, mostly because they usually parallel something basic in the average kitchen that already does the trick. The Wish List deserves consideration, because its items will dramatically limit the time spent in preparing food that can also be made using your basic equipment. If you're serious about making your kitchen time quick and painless, consider splurging. Otherwise, just stick with the Must-Haves.

The total cost of upgrading your kitchen equipment should never exceed, at maximum, a few hundred dollars, especially if you've already got some of these tools and you're starting first with the basics. Shop around. Prices for an item can vary widely, so research first before you buy.

This list assumes that your kitchen already contains an oven with a broiler and a good selection of pots, pans, and knives. More than anything else, a high-quality sharp knife, a heavy-bottomed, high-capacity skillet (approximately 12 inches in diameter and at least 2 inches deep, preferably in cast iron), and a well-made, high-capacity 12-quart stockpot or Dutch oven are necessities for any kitchen.

A final word on typical kitchen gear: Brazilians don't generally use microwaves. Neither do I. While I appreciate that a microwave can be an excellent time-saving appliance to defrost frozen items, cooking in it often yields rubbery meals with no texture, so I stay away from them and leave everything to my ancient but fantastic oven, my toaster oven with rotisserie, and my four-burner stove. If I need to defrost something, I make a note to take it out of the freezer the night before and pop it in to the fridge to defrost overnight.

MUST-HAVE KITCHEN TOOLS

Alligator chopper. Brazilian food requires a lot of diced onion, as well as peppers and other vegetables. Nothing could be more tedious and time consuming than chopping an onion. That's why the Alligator chopper, which dices half an onion in one swift motion, is such a great tool in the kitchen. Forget about tears. Find it for under thirty dollars.

Blender. Don't skimp on this one. Make it a blender of high quality. You will be making a lot of smoothies, so it pays to find a sturdy model whose blades won't bend and whose liquid receptacle—make sure it's glass and not plastic—won't crack or split. To double up on utility, you can buy a good-quality model that also has a food processor attachment. Oster makes a pretty good one for under fifty dollars. (See also **Hand blender**.)

Coffee grinder. Not for coffee, but for nuts, dried shrimp, and other items that need to be rendered to powder for Brazilian recipes. Braun makes great mini-grinders for less than twenty dollars.

Food storage containers. You'll need several of these in various sizes and shapes for storing sauces, diced vegetables, leftovers, cakes, and puddings, or for marinating meats. Make sure to get at least three large, deep-bottomed tubs (approximately 12 inches in diameter and 6 inches deep) to hold cakes or pies. You'll also need small (approximately 4 cups in volume) and medium-size (approximately 6-cup or 8-cup) containers. Beware of Tupperware and its ilk: Plastic can be very reactive—even toxic—with food, especially acidic liquids, which feature in a lot of Brazilian cuisine, so be clever and frugal. Glass containers that you would otherwise throw away (peanut butter, pickle, and condiment jars, wine bottles) can be cleaned, sterilized in boiling water, and recycled as containers. Look through your glass and nonreactive metal baking dishes and mixing bowls and try to use those to hold your food. Avoid using plastic except for nonliquid items. With the money you save in recycling your glass, buy a few vacuum stoppers for the wine bottles.

Hand blender. When you need to puree a soup or a sauce while it's still in the stockpot, a hand blender makes the process quicker and easier than decanting it into a separate blender. Hand blenders also clean up quickly and easily. They're also invaluable for reconstituting sauces that may be separating under heat. I use Braun's hand blender products in my kitchen, and their excellent Multiquick Deluxe Hand Blender and Chopper also comes with whip and food processor attachments—more value for your money at around twenty-five dollars. The professional version of this set, at eighty dollars, is a full-power blender and food processor, thereby obviating the need to buy separate blenders or food processors.

Mandoline. As with the blender, don't skimp on the quality of a mandoline by going on price alone, otherwise you'll lose a finger, or worse. Mandolines are very sharp and potentially very dangerous when you're trying to work quickly, so find a sturdy one that allows you to slice and julienne at top speed. For kitchen novices and pros alike, I think

Swissmar Borner's V-Slicer Plus is the best all-round model at a very reasonable price, usually under thirty-five dollars. For kitchen whizzes used to handling mandolines, I like Dean and Deluca's Super Benriner at under seventy dollars.

Pan. Perhaps you have lots of cheap skillets and saucepans taking up space. Maybe it's time to downsize and invest in one good, 12-inch diameter skillet with at least a 2-inch depth. The deeper the pan, the more versatile, as you can use the pan not only for frying but also for making sauces. If you can afford cast iron, splurge. A well-seasoned cast-iron pan lasts longer, conducts heat much more effectively, and requires less oil to cook food since proper seasoning creates a virtually nonstick surface. You can also place cast-iron pans into ovens to roast and finish foods cooked on the stove.

Pudding molds or ramekins. Brazilians love their puddings. Puddings are not only easy to make, they can be desserts that even people who need to watch their weight can eat—especially since a mold allows you to maintain portion control over individual servings. If you don't already have these in your kitchen, you'll need individual molds to prepare some of the program's recipes. Hunt down cheap, decorative ovenproof molds from restaurant supply houses.

Salad and herb spinner. You'll be cleaning and rinsing a lot of leaves and vegetables, so make your life easier by purchasing a good spinner. I'm a big fan of OXO Good Grips Salad spinners because they clean and also serve as storage and crisping containers for the rinsed and dried veggies. Zyliss makes good ones, too. Find one for under twenty dollars.

Sharp knife. Invest in a high-quality multipurpose knife. These are expensive, but they'll last longer and make kitchen preparation easier. I prefer Santoku knives for their range of use and the best of the lot is the Shun Classic 6.5-inch knife by Kai. Expect to pay a little under a hundred dollars for the knife and a sharpening stone to preserve the blade for a lifetime.

Silicon pastry brush. To "paint" flavored sauces onto grilled meats to control portion size, a silicon pastry brush makes all the difference. They don't react to hot sauces and they are easy to clean. You can usually find decent ones for well under ten dollars.

Steamer. Small and cheap, steamers may be made of metal or bamboo. Metal lasts longer—provided the metal is galvanized—but bamboo steamers are often less expensive

(I can get them in New York's Chinatown for less than five dollars for a large one). The metal steamers' advantage lies in how they collapse to a small shape that takes up less storage room, which may be a requirement for apartment dwellers with tiny kitchens.

Stockpot. A good kitchen should always contain a 12-quart heavy stockpot (or a Dutch oven) for preparing soups, stews, and sauces. Avoid flimsy aluminum pots that dent easily or whose coating flakes off.

Vegetable julienne peeler. When you need a small amount of julienned carrot, zucchini, or potato, a sturdy julienne peeler can render strips from an entire vegetable in less than 30 seconds, with no equipment to clean. OXO Good Grips makes the best one I've ever used, for under fifteen dollars.

WISH-LIST KITCHEN TOOLS

Apple corer. The BBBP uses a lot of apples. Coring them is a time-stealer, so a device that can core and split the apple into slices in one swift motion is a neat gadget to have in the kitchen. You could slice around the core with a mandoline, but you need deft hands to achieve that quickly. A corer's not a necessity, but it helps. OXO Good Grips comes through again with a cheap yet superlatively designed product for around five dollars.

Food processor. If you've splashed out on Must-Have tools without food processor attachments, consider getting one at some point. For chopping large amounts of vegetables, and other chores, it does save on time. Good ones can be found for under seventy dollars.

Garlic press. Most of the time, I simply crush several cloves simultaneously by smashing them under the blade of a cleaver and then giving them a quick chop. But I also use a flat, heavy rock from my garden to crush them in one blow. You could probably do the same. A garlic press is not a necessity, but if you can't apply sufficient force, OXO Good Grips makes a nice press, for under ten dollars, that extracts more garlic than others I've used.

George Foreman Champ Grill. Odds are you already have one of these at home, just based on the sheer number of these little babies sold. The sales volume is justified: It grills food for up to two people evenly, quickly, and allows the fat to run off. You could use a grill pan, or work with your oven broiler, but the George Foreman grills do it quicker and better. It's a great, well-designed product at a good price—usually under twenty dollars.

Mezzaluna. You'll be preparing a lot of minced herbs and vegetables. You could do this with two knives or in a food processor (though you risk crushing herbs this way); a mezzaluna (a two-handled wood chopper) is simply a better tool for mincing herb mixtures. It chops just about anything quickly and ergonomically—which helps if you don't have enough dexterity or strength to manipulate other utensils. You can find good ones for under thirty dollars.

Rice cooker. Sure, you could just boil water in a stockpot and cook the rice. Or you can put it in a rice cooker in the morning before you go to work and have it hot and ready by the time you're back. Not necessary, but it does save a lot of time when rice is on the menu. While the BBBP does not emphasize rice on a daily basis, it features it often enough that a rice cooker can be a very useful kitchen device to have. I swear by my Zojirushi 5-cup rice cooker, priced at under eighty dollars. But the company, which I believe makes the best rice cookers on the market, also offers a smaller cooker for under forty dollars, too.

Toaster oven with rotisserie function. If you don't already have a toaster oven, consider getting a dual-function oven with a rotisserie feature. Rotisseries are a godsend in the kitchen because they allow you to prepare perfectly roasted meat far more easily, cleanly, and effectively than in conventional ovens. Just slide a marinated chicken (or pork loin, or beef roast, or whatever else you prefer) onto the spit, turn it on, and walk away. A little over an hour later you have a fragrantly crisp and juicy bird. I have a model by Tefal that gets used at least once a week for roast dinners. It's one of my favorite kitchen items and, at a hundred and fifty dollars, not bargain-basement cheap, but not outrageous, either.

Zesting grater. You'll be zesting a lot of citrus fruits for recipes, so while a plain old grater should be okay, you'll get more shapely shreds out of a zester. If not handled properly, sharp zesters can be as dangerous as they are stylish. I especially like the Microplane zesters, which cost well under ten dollars.

3

Thirty Days the Brazilian Way

THE BRAZILIAN BIKINI BODY PROGRAM pairs the best of Brazilian cuisine with an exercise program that can be incorporated into anyone's lifestyle. Apply a *jeitinho*, or a bit of pragmatic attitude to this regimen and you'll sail past roadblocks or problems that may emerge.

For thirty days, your breakfast, lunch, and dinner will be composed of the very Brazilian flavors of key superfoods. A breakfast made from antioxidant-packed *açaí* forms the cornerstone of your daily meals; lunches and dinners build on that by mixing and matching basic, easy-to-prepare sauces that can be dabbed in small amounts on marinated lean meats and fish for maximum flavor. Nuts and legumes and vegetables in the form of soups and salads round out a program that emphasizes easy and healthy home cooking. Desserts, in portions that offer a few small but sweet mouthfuls, offer a counterpoint to meals and can prevent you from tipping over into bad habits due to deprivation. To keep you on a virtuous track, the program makes strategic use of left-overs, so you don't waste food.

Fueled by such wholesome and tasty meals, you'll be ready to take on the exercise program, composed of three workouts: the Mini Workout (10 minutes), the Half-Hour Workout, and the Full-Hour Workout. Complete information on each of the workouts can be found in chapter 5. To keep track of your progress, you can use the workout logs on page 250.

So how do you apply a *jeitinho*? First, start the program on a Sunday. That way, you'll have ample time to shop and prepare foods for the week. Tear out, or make copies of, the weekly shopping lists found on pages 240–49. Then follow the calendar on pages 235–39 that lays out the food preparation needed to take you through the thirty days as efficiently as possible. Second, don't freak out if you can't find an ingredient or don't want to eat a particular food. Relax and substitute. Don't like red meat? Try turkey or chicken. Vegetarian? Use soy protein instead. Finicky? Pick out what you like and improvise with the rest. Just try to remember to keep your improvisations within the framework of a solid breakfast; simple sauces "painted" on lean, marinated meats; and a good mix of nuts, beans, and vegetables.

Stick to this program to the best of your ability, and you'll be able to celebrate the changes in your body. To that end, the thirty-day plan includes three party suggestions so you can show off your new cooking skills and share some of the fabulous food with your family and friends. After all, as every Brazilian knows, life's no fun without parties.

WEEK 1

DAY 1 / SUNDAY

MENU

Breakfast: Automatic Pilot
Late lunch/early dinner: Brazilian Chicken Pot Pie;
Classic Brazilian Salad; Nut-Crusted Apple Pie

Midmorning snack: Crunchy Nuts with Soy
Midafternoon snack: Romeo and Juliet

EXERCISE

Mini workout: See page 183

NOTE: *The BBBP's Saturday and Sunday meals are designed for all-day eating so that you only have to cook once. Try to organize your meals around social gatherings. Invite friends or family to share big, laid-back feasts—think of these festive meals as late brunches. Plan to have your big meal in the midafternoon, around three P.M. If you're a bit hungry in the evening, have a light meal of what you made for lunch no later than eight P.M.*

DAY 2 / MONDAY

MENU

Breakfast: Automatic Pilot
Lunch: Shrimp Mini-Pie (or Chicken Pot Pie
leftovers); Chickpea Salad
Dinner: Roasted Fish with Shrimp Sauce; Seaweed
Rice; Nut-Crusted Apple Pie

Midmorning snack: Crunchy Nuts with Chile and
Lime
Midafternoon snack: Vitamina Green

EXERCISE

Mini Workout: Twice—in the morning after you get up and again after work. See page 183.

DAY 3 / TUESDAY

MENU

Breakfast: Automatic Pilot
Lunch: Palm Heart Soup; Chickpea Salad
Dinner: Grilled Chicken with Coriander-Garlic
Sauce; Watercress Salad; Nut-Crusted Apple Pie

Midmorning snack: Cold Maté with Lime
Midafternoon snack: Coconut Water

EXERCISE

Mini Workout: Once—in the morning after getting up. See page 183.
Half-Hour Workout: Once—in the evening after work. See page 183.

DAY 4 / WEDNESDAY

MENU

Breakfast: Automatic Pilot
Lunch: Chicken Sandwich/Wrap; Palm Heart Soup;
    Classic Brazilian Salad
Dinner: Beef with Onions; Black Bean Salad; Fruit
    Salad

Midmorning snack: Crunchy Nuts with Soy
Midafternoon snack: Vitamina Red

EXERCISE

Full-Hour Workout: See page 184.

DAY 5 / THURSDAY

MENU

Breakfast: Automatic Pilot
Lunch: Shrimp Pie; Watercress Salad
Dinner: Brazilian Chicken Stroganoff; Rice with
    Broccoli; Fruit Salad

Midmorning snack: Romeo and Juliet
Midafternoon snack: Crunchy Nuts with Chile and
    Lime

EXERCISE

Mini Workout: Twice—in the morning after you get up and again after work. See page 183.

DAY 6 / FRIDAY

MENU

Breakfast: Super C Bomb
Late Lunch: Palm Heart Soup; Natural
    Sandwich/Wrap
Dinner: Shrimp and Egg Bake; Black Bean Salad;
    Fruit Salad

Midmorning snack: Vitamina Yellow
Midafternoon snack: Coconut Water

EXERCISE

Full-Hour Workout: See page 184.

DAY 7 / SATURDAY

MENU

Breakfast: Automatic Pilot
Late lunch/early dinner: Wagoner's Rice; Spinach
    Salad; Prune Compote

Midmorning snack: Coconut Water
Midafternoon snack: Romeo and Juliet

EXERCISE

Half-Hour Workout: See page 183.

NOTE: *Saturday is your shop-and-chop day. The bulk of the food preparation work takes place over the weekend so that you'll have only minimal work to do during weekdays, when you'll be less inclined to be in the kitchen.*

WEEK 2

DAY 8 / SUNDAY

MENU

Breakfast: Automatic Pilot
Late lunch/early dinner: Oxtail and Watercress Stew; Potatoes with Nori; Coconut Flan with Prune Compote

Midmorning snack: Cold Maté with Lime
Midafternoon snack: Vitamina Green

EXERCISE
Full-Hour Workout: See page 184.

NOTE: *Oxtail stew is a very rich meal, so aim to eat this late lunch a little earlier, closer to midday. If you are squeamish about oxtail, consider substituting beef short ribs instead. You can have the Vitamina as your evening meal if you're not hungry enough in the late afternoon to drink it.*

DAY 9 / MONDAY

MENU

Breakfast: Vitamina Yellow
Lunch: Miso Soup; Lentil Salad
Dinner: Fried Fish; Broccoli and Cauliflower with Spinach Sauce; Coconut Flan and Prune Compote

Midmorning snack: Romeo and Juliet
Midafternoon snack: Honey-Nut Crumble

EXERCISE
Mini Workout: Twice—in the morning after you get up and again after work. See page 183.

DAY 10 / TUESDAY

MENU

Breakfast: Automatic Pilot
Lunch: Tuna Salad; Watercress Salad
Dinner: Roast Pork Loin; Lentil Salad; Coconut Flan and Prune Compote

Midmorning snack: Coconut Water
Midafternoon snack: Vitamina Green

EXERCISE
Mini Workout: Once—in the morning after getting up. See page 183.
Half-Hour Workout: Once—in the evening after work. See page 183.

DAY 11 / WEDNESDAY

MENU

Breakfast: Automatic Pilot
Lunch: Roast Pork Loin Sandwiches/Wraps with
　Spinach Sauce; Classic Brazilian Salad
Dinner: Grilled Turkey Breast with Nutty Mango
　Vinaigrette; Palm Heart Salad; Brazilian Fudge
　Balls

Midmorning snack: Cold Maté with Lime
Midafternoon snack: Vitamina Red

EXERCISE

Full-Hour Workout: See page 184.

DAY 12 / THURSDAY

MENU

Breakfast: Automatic Pilot
Lunch: Miso Soup; Turkey Sandwich/Wrap with
　Vinaigrette
Dinner: Roasted Meatballs; Black Bean Puree;
　Classic Brazilian Salad; Brazilian Fudge Balls

Midmorning snack: Honey-Nut Crumble
Midafternoon snack: Vitamina Yellow

EXERCISE

Mini Workout: Twice—in the morning after you get up and again after work. See page 183.

DAY 13 / FRIDAY

MENU

Breakfast: Super C bomb
Lunch: Falafel; Watercress Salad
Dinner: Cashew-Crusted Baked Fish with Lime
　Sauce; Yucca Fries; Kale, Minas Style; Brazilian
　Fudge Balls

Midmorning snack: Romeo and Juliet
Midafternoon snack: Roasted Meatball

EXERCISE

Full-Hour Workout: See page 184.

DAY 14 / SATURDAY

MENU

Breakfast: Automatic Pilot
Late lunch/early dinner: Brazilian Chicken Soup with
　Rice; Efó; Malted Milk Panna Cotta

Midmorning snack: Guaraná
Midafternoon snack: Roasted Meatball

EXERCISE

Half-Hour Workout: See page 183.

NOTE: *As with all Saturday and Sunday late lunch/early dinner all-day meals, you can have small portions of the dishes and graze on them throughout the day, if you don't fancy having one large midday meal.*

WEEK 3

DAY 15 / SUNDAY

MENU

Breakfast: Automatic Pilot

Late lunch/early dinner: Cozido; Arugula Sauce; Chunky Vinaigrette; Malted Milk Panna Cotta

Midmorning snack: Crunchy Nuts with Soy

Midafternoon snack: Vitamina Green

EXERCISE

Full-Hour Workout: See page 184.

NOTE: Cozido *has several components which make it a great all-day meal. Have the meat and vegetables earlier in the day as your larger meal. Then have the spiced broth the dish makes, and some more vegetables, for your smaller meal later in the day.*

DAY 16 / MONDAY

MENU

Breakfast: Automatic Pilot

Lunch: Sausage and Beef Sandwiches/Wraps with either Nutty Mango Vinaigrette or Arugula Sauce; Hijiki Salad

Dinner: Grilled Chicken with Arugula Sauce; Rice with Broccoli; Malted Milk Panna Cotta

Midmorning snack: Romeo and Juliet

Midafternoon snack: Honey-Nut Crumble

EXERCISE

Mini Workout: Twice—in the morning after you get up and again after work. See page 183.

DAY 17 / TUESDAY

MENU

Breakfast: Vitamina Yellow

Lunch: Watercress Soup; Chicken Sandwich/Wrap with Coriander-Garlic Sauce

Dinner: Grilled Steak with Chunky Vinaigrette; Hijiki Salad; Wobbly Marias

Midmorning snack: Crunchy Nuts with Chile and Lime

Midafternoon snack: Coconut Water

EXERCISE

Mini Workout: Once—in the morning after getting up. See page 183.

Half-Hour Workout: Once—in the evening after work. See page 183.

DAY 18 / WEDNESDAY

MENU

Breakfast: Automatic Pilot
Lunch: Bauru Sandwich/Wrap; Classic Brazilian
 Salad
Dinner: Watercress Soup; Tuna Salad; Wobbly Marias

Midmorning snack: Swiss Lemonade
Midafternoon snack: Crunchy Nuts with Soy

EXERCISE

Full-Hour Workout: See page 184.

DAY 19 / THURSDAY

MENU

Breakfast: Super C bomb
Lunch: Watercress Soup; Gnocchi with Arugula Sauce
Dinner: Garlic Chicken; Palm Heart Salad; Wobbly
 Marias

Midmorning snack: Coconut Water
Midafternoon snack: Romeo and Juliet

EXERCISE

Mini Workout: Once—in the morning after getting up. See page 183.
Half-Hour Workout: Once—in the evening after work. See page 183.

DAY 20 / FRIDAY

MENU

Breakfast: Automatic Pilot
Lunch: Eggplant Salad
Dinner: Sushi Party—Miso Soup; Nigiri Sushi and
 Sashimi; Hijiki Salad; Pumpkin Tartlets

Midmorning snack: Honey-Nut Crumble
Midafternoon snack: Coconut Water

EXERCISE

Mini Workout: Twice—in the morning after you get up and again after work. See page 183.

DAY 21 / SATURDAY

MENU

Breakfast: Automatic Pilot
Late Lunch/Early Dinner: Acarajé; Moqueca; Açaí-
 Strawberry Pudding

Midmorning Snack: Guaraná
Midafternoon Snack: Vitamina Green

EXERCISE

Half-Hour Workout: See page 183.

NOTE: *This all-day Bahian menu is tasty, but very rich. Acarajé is a fried treat, so remember not to overindulge. Leave enough room for the moqueca stew and the pudding dessert. As before, if you weren't hungry enough in the late afternoon for your Vitamina, have it for your last meal of the day later on closer to the dinnertime—or leave it out altogether if you feel satisfied by the main meal.*

WEEK 4

DAY 22 / SUNDAY

MENU

Breakfast: Automatic Pilot
Late lunch/early dinner: BBQ Party—Stuffed Crab
    Shells; Churrasco; Chunky Vinaigrette;
    Watercress Sauce; Classic Brazilian Salad;
    Batida; Açaí-Strawberry Pudding

Midmorning snack: Romeo and Juliet
Midafternoon snack: Vitamina Yellow

EXERCISE

Full-Hour Workout: See page 184.

NOTE: *The BBQ party is a large buffet. Graze on the different dishes throughout the day and try not to eat too much of any one thing. Limit your intake of alcoholic cocktails and balance them against how much dessert you eat.*

DAY 23 / MONDAY

MENU

Breakfast: Automatic Pilot
Lunch: Black Bean Soup; Palm Heart Salad
Dinner: Brazilian Mincemeat; Cabbage Salad;
    Seaweed Rice; Açaí-Strawberry Pudding

Midmorning snack: Coconut Water
Midafternoon snack: Crunchy Nuts with Chili and
    Lime

EXERCISE

Full-Hour Workout: See page 184.

DAY 24 / TUESDAY

MENU

Breakfast: Automatic Pilot
Lunch: Roast Zucchini Stuffed with Brazilian
    Mincemeat; Cabbage Salad
Dinner: Roast Chicken with Vegetables; Spinach
    Salad; Coconut-Tapioca Pudding

Midmorning snack: Romeo and Juliet
Midafternoon snack: Vitamina Red

EXERCISE

Mini Workout: Once—in the morning after getting up. See page 183.
Half-Hour Workout: Once—in the evening after work. See page 183.

DAY 25 / WEDNESDAY

MENU

Breakfast: Automatic Pilot
Lunch: Chicken Sandwiches/Wraps with either
    Watercress or Limacello Vinaigrette; Classic
    Brazilian Salad

Midmorning snack: Coconut Water
Midafternoon snack: Honey-Nut Crumble

Dinner: Black Bean Soup; Grilled Steak with either
    Anchovy Sauce or Gorgonzola Sauce; Kale,
    Minas Style; Coconut-Tapioca Pudding

EXERCISE
Half-Hour Workout: See page 183.

DAY 26 / THURSDAY

MENU

Breakfast: Super C bomb
Lunch: Black Bean Soup; Bauru Sandwich/Wrap
Dinner: Sautéed Turkey Breast with either
    Gorgonzola Sauce or Anchovy Sauce;
    Spinach Salad; Coconut-Tapioca Pudding

Midmorning snack: Coconut Water
Midafternoon snack: Vitamina Green

EXERCISE
Mini Workout: Once—in the morning after getting up. See page 183.
Half-Hour Workout: Once—in the evening after work. See page 183.

DAY 27 / FRIDAY

MENU

Breakfast: Automatic Pilot
Lunch: Acarajé with Acarajé Sauce; Watercress Salad
Dinner: Vatapá; Rice with Broccoli; Coconut-
    Tapioca Pudding

Midmorning snack: Romeo and Juliet
Midafternoon snack: Coconut Water

EXERCISE
Full-Hour Workout: See page 184.

DAY 28 / SATURDAY

MENU

Breakfast: Automatic Pilot
Late lunch/early dinner: Cod Gomes de Sá;
    Watercress Salad; Orange Cake

Midmorning snack: Honey-Nut Crumble
Midafternoon snack: Vitamina Yellow

EXERCISE
Full-Hour Workout: See page 184.

NOTE: *The cod can be eaten hot or cold, and it stores well. As with other Saturday and Sunday meals, you can pick at it throughout the day. Try having the cod hot for your midday meal, then eat it cold for the last small meal of the day.*

WEEK 5

DAY 29 / SUNDAY

MENU

Breakfast: Automatic Pilot

Late lunch/early dinner: *Feijoada* Party—Salt Cod
    Fritters; Cheese Rolls; Black Bean and Meat
    Stew; Kale, Minas Style; Rice with Broccoli;
    Pepper Sauce; Quentão; Caipirinha; the
    Paulistano; Caipirissima; Orange Cake

Midmorning snack: Coconut Water

EXERCISE

Full-Hour Workout: See page 184.

NOTE: *Eat* feijoada *closer to noon. You'll need the better part of the day to digest this heavy meal. Try to plan your workout for late in the afternoon, at least three hours after you've eaten. As before, watch your alcohol intake and balance that against your consumption of treats like fritters, cheese rolls, and cake. It's a party, but be sensible.*

DAY 30 / MONDAY

MENU

Breakfast: Automatic Pilot

Lunch: Caldo Verde

Dinner: Ximxim de Galinha; Classic Brazilian Salad;
    Orange Cake

Midmorning snack: Crunchy Nuts with Soy

Midafternoon snack: Coconut Water

EXERCISE

Mini Workout: Twice—in the morning after you get up and again after work. See page 183.

SETTING THE SCENE WHILE SETTING THE TABLE

As you prepare these delicious foods, let the sounds of Brazil accompany you in your kitchen and to the dining table.

Dining Music: Five Critical Brazilian Bossa Nova Songs

1. "Chega de Saudade" (No More Blues): Tom Jobim/Vinícius de Moraes
2. "Desafinado" (Off Key): Tom Jobim/Newton Mendonça
3. "Garota de Ipanema" (Girl from Ipanema): Tom Jobim/Vinícius de Moraes
4. "Insensatez" (How Insensitive): Tom Jobim/Vinícius de Moraes
5. "Samba de Uma Nota So" (One-Note Samba): Tom Jobim/Newton Mendonça

Six Critical Brazilian Composers

1. Gilberto Gil
2. João Gilberto
3. Tom Jobim
4. Baden Powell
5. Caetano Veloso
6. Heitor Villa-Lobos

4

Come! ("Eat!"): The Recipes

THE FOLLOWING RECIPES provide an authentic taste of Brazil. A few of these are classics I've gathered from the lovingly preserved recipe boxes belonging to relatives and friends; most are versions I've developed from observation and years of kitchen work; and some are recipes I've created from putting together the basic Brazilian building blocks of ingredients. Remember to watch your portion sizes, but don't be afraid to substitute or add or subtract certain ingredients according to your dietary or taste preferences. Enjoy!

• • •

DRINKS/COCKTAILS

Automatic Pilot
(In Homage to Big Nectar)

If you change one thing in your life, make it this: Drink the Automatic Pilot as your daily breakfast. Quick and easy to prepare, a nutritious Automatic Pilot packs the antioxidant punch of açaí, along with the protein from soy milk and peanut butter. It may come in shake form, but this drink feels like a meal: The fiber in both the banana and the açaí ensure that you will stay full until lunch. Your body will burn the calories more efficiently over time, thanks to the right balance of fat, protein, sugar, and carbohydrates. More important, the complex flavors of chocolate, berry, peanut, and banana combine to make this an appealingly sweet treat to "break the fast" of sleep. This recipe takes its name from a drink named Piloto Automatico served at my favorite juice bar in Rio, Big Nectar—a magnet for the local surfers and athletes who love Big Nectar's fruit smoothies. My recipe departs from the original by using soy milk and leaving out a big dose of honey, resulting in less sugar and more protein.

1 (3.5-ounce) packet frozen *açaí* pulp (preferably pre-sweetened and infused
    with *guaraná*)
1 banana
¼ cup vanilla soy milk
1 teaspoon peanut butter (I prefer crunchy, but smooth works, too—or
    use ¼ cup unsalted peanuts)

Place all ingredients in a blender and whip until smooth. Pour into a 10-ounce (or larger) glass and enjoy.

Servings: 1
Preparation time: 5 minutes or less

Super C Bomb
(In Homage to Big Nectar)

Here's a recipe modeled on another Big Nectar smoothie called "Super C Bomba." If you're looking for an immune system booster, try this citric, vitamin C–loaded shake. The flavor base is acerola, a tart, cherry-like tropical fruit also known as the "Barbados cherry." Strawberries and orange juice make this version sweeter than Big Nectar's; they help to balance acerola's tang, while adding calcium and other minerals to the mix. If you still find this a bit too mouth-puckering, add no more than a teaspoon of honey or Splenda. Otherwise, you can just leave out the extra sweetener. Drink this when you feel a bit rundown or are experiencing the early symptoms of a cold or flu.

> 1 (3.5-ounce) packet or ½ cup frozen acerola pulp
> ¾ cup orange juice
> ½ cup fresh or frozen strawberries
> ¼ cup water
> 1 teaspoon honey or Splenda, if desired

Place all ingredients in a blender and whip until smooth.

Servings: 1
Preparation time: 5 minutes or less

Vitaminas

In Brazil, vitaminas *are smoothies made with milk or yogurt. I actually prefer the taste of soy milk—as well as its protein and phytoestrogens—to that of the real thing. You can always, however, use skim milk if you prefer it to soy. These three color-coded shakes can cure what ails you: Go Green when you've missed eating lettuces and leaves; yield to Yellow when you're stressed, tired, or sick and need a jolt to the immune system; and stop and reach for Red when you've consumed too many heavy, creamy meals.*

Vitamina Green

> 2 stalks celery
> ½ apple, cored
> 1 handful of parsley
> ½ pear, cored
> ¼ cup plain soy milk

Place all ingredients in a blender and whip until smooth.

Servings: 1
Preparation time: 5 minutes or less

Vitamina Yellow

> ½ cup frozen mango
> Juice of 1 lemon
> ½ cup orange juice
> ¼ cup vanilla soy milk

Place all ingredients in a blender and whip until smooth.

Servings: 1
Preparation time: 5 minutes or less

Vitamina Red

½ apple, cored
½ cup strawberries
½ cup blueberries
¼ cup vanilla soy milk

Place all ingredients in a blender and whip until smooth.

Servings: 1
Preparation time: 5 minutes or less

Swiss Lemonade
(Limonada Suiça)

Hot weather calls for generous glasses of cool, fizzy lemonade. In Brazil, lemonade is made with limes, which are more common than lemons. This drink may be Swiss in name, but the tart freshness of lime gives it a Brazilian flair.

Juice of 1 lime
1 cup seltzer water
½ cup crushed ice
1 teaspoon Splenda or 5 drops stevia

Mix all the ingredients and pour into a tall glass.

Servings: 1
Preparation time: 5 minutes or less

Maté with Lime
(Matte com Limão)

Matte [MAH-chee] is sold in the United States as yerba maté tea, often found in health food stores or organic markets. While maté is used throughout South America as a potent tea with antioxidant properties, I find the way it is sold in Brazil far more charming. On the beaches of Brazil, maté hawkers carry a gleaming steel drum of cold maté tea that pours out through a delicate spigot and into a cup garnished with a slice of lime. Those steel drums of cold tea, dewy with condensation and sporting the lion-head mascot of the Matte Leão brand (Brazil's most popular maté), do as much to refresh by their mere sight as do their contents. Maté contains some caffeine (though not as much as coffee), so watch your intake, and be sure to drink it early in the day; drinking maté in the evening can keep you awake and prevent you from getting enough rest.

> **1 tea bag maté tea**
> **Juice of ½ lime**
> **1 teaspoon Splenda or 5 drops stevia**

Brew the tea and let it steep for 3 minutes. Add the sweetener. This can be drunk hot or cold.

Servings: 1
Preparation time: 5 minutes or less

Traditional Caipirinha

Ah, Brazil's national cocktail—so memorable, so tasty, and so potent. And such a catalyst for debate among cocktail connoisseurs, mostly over botched preparations that confuse it with Cuba's minty mojitos. A caipirinha's chief attraction is its ability to seduce its swillers with its light, refreshing taste, then quickly reduce them to rubber-legged blobs of protoplasm. How else could tourists in Brazil become such good samba dancers so quickly upon their arrival? Make no mistake: Cachaça, the liquor that forms the base of the cocktail, is rocket fuel made from sugarcane and about as alcoholic as grain-based spirits—usually 40 to 50 percent alcohol by volume or around 80 proof. Caipirinhas are indispensable at Brazilian parties, feijoada or churrasco feasts, or at just about any social gathering. A little goes a long way; so drink these in moderation. Be creative with the caipirinha recipe by adding different spirits to make caipiroskas *(using vodka) and* caipirissimas *(using Brazilian rum), or add tart tropical juices like passion fruit to the* cachaça *recipe for a Brazilian twist on the original cocktail recipe.*

1 lime, quartered
1 teaspoon sugar
½ cup crushed ice
4 tablespoons *cachaça*

Squeeze the juice of two of the lime quarters into a wide-mouthed glass. Place one of the lime quarters at the bottom of the glass and add the sugar. Using a wooden spoon or other wooden implement, muddle the lime and sugar until a smooth paste is achieved. Add the ice and pour the *cachaça* into the glass. Thoroughly mix all the ingredients. Serve garnished with the last lime quarter.

Servings: 1
Preparation time: 5 minutes or less

VARIATION: **Caipiroska**
Use the Caipirinha recipe, but substitute 4 tablespoons of high-quality vodka for *cachaça*.

Caipirissima

Try this caipirinha *made with Brazilian rum. Oronoco is the best one available in the United States.*

1 lime, quartered
1.5 ounces high-quality Brazilian white rum, preferably Oronoco
1 teaspoon sugar
Splash of lime juice
1 stalk sugarcane, for garnish

Muddle the lime wedges in a shaker. Add the rum, sugar, and lime juice. Shake with ice. Strain the contents into a martini glass and garnish with the sugarcane stalk.

Servings: 1
Preparation time: 5 minutes or less

VICENTE BASTOS RIBEIRO

Master distiller and businessman Bastos Ribeiro's family farm, the Fazenda Soledade, in Rio de Janeiro state, produces Brazil's most recognized premium *cachaças* and rums. He is also a member of BNG2, a nongovernmental organization that backs environmentall friendly practices and the preservation of natural resources. Bastos Ribeiro passionately supports sustainable farming techniques and local growers.

I like to think of myself as a Brazilian analogue to a French vintner, using sugarcane like the finest varietal grapes. To me, as to any serious farmers who love their land and what it can produce, the terroir [soil] is an obsession. I spend a lot of time in the outdoors, appreciating the land that allows me to pursue my passion for making fine spirits, and I try to put that appreciation right back into the soil. We follow the strictest environmental growing methods so as not to disturb the land. Conservation and recycling are a constant preoccupation for me.

I really enjoy staying active. I used to work out at a gym, but that didn't satisfy me at all. Then I hurt my neck and had to give up traditional workouts. I wanted to find something more harmonious, so I thought I would give Pilates a try. I fell in love with it from the very first time. I've been doing it for over two years now, and I feel so great. I'm so much more balanced and "in" my body, which I really need. I have a very heavy schedule, going back and forth between the farm and my business offices in Rio, and Pilates helps me restore my sense of strength and calm. I do it three times a week, and I think you could say I'm hooked.

I live a very eclectic life—or lives. Sometimes I'll be out doing business and socializing with bankers, sometimes I'll hang out with musicians. I love to go see rock bands, even now at fifty-five years old! I have this theory of averages—you have to balance out being good and being indulgent, so that you can have both. I love to cook and eat well, I'm passionate about French gastronomy and I'm very into wine. I had to find a jeitinho to eat better so that I wasn't always eating rich food. So I found a great macrobiotic restaurant in downtown Rio. Now I break my day up into distinct parts. I'll eat healthy macrobiotic food at lunchtime, which then allows me to go out with friends to have evening meals with fine wines. I can't always manage this balance, but I do my best.

The Paulistano

Natives of São Paulo savor this popular cocktail in the city's hottest late-night clubs.

3 lime wedges
1.5 ounces Oronoco rum
Mint leaves
1 ounce pineapple juice
Splash of orange Cognac
1 stalk sugarcane, for garnish

Muddle the lime wedges in a shaker. Add the rum, mint, pineapple juice, and orange Cognac. Shake with ice. Strain into a martini glass and garnish with the sugarcane stalk.

Servings: 1
Preparation time: 5 minutes or less

Quentão

This cocktail is similar to warmed, spirit-based drinks such as hot toddies, Scandinavian glogg, or hot buttered rum. While those drinks tend to be served on frigid nights, this libation from the region of São Paulo—served on St. John's Day, the twenty-fourth of June, in Brazil's winter—quenches thirsts when the coldest temperatures waver around 60°F.

1 thimble-size piece fresh ginger, shredded
2 cinnamon sticks
¼ teaspoon grated nutmeg
2 cloves
½ cup sugar or Splenda
1 cup water
1 cup *cachaça*
1 lime, sliced finely, for garnish

Place the ginger, cinnamon, nutmeg, cloves, sugar, and water in a saucepan. Bring to a boil, then strain through a fine colander, reserving the cinnamon sticks. Add the *cachaça* to the liquid and serve hot, garnished with the cinnamon sticks and lime slices.

Servings: 4
Preparation time: 10 minutes or less

Batidas

When I was a child, my parents' cocktail parties evoked a real sense of anticipation: What should be worn, which menu would be prepared, and most of all, what kinds of batidas would be served. A batida is an adult's milkshake (batida means "beaten" in Portuguese). Coconut milk serves as the base to which cachaça, rum, and all sorts of fruits and flavors—even peanut butter!—are added. My father considered himself a batida wizard and would experiment like a Nobel Prize–winning chemist, slipping my sister and me a few tastes here and there if we bugged him enough on a special occasion. In general, my sister and I were restricted to nonalcoholic versions of these sweet, frothy drinks as a very rare treat. In Brazil, coconut, passion fruit, and, yes, peanut butter batidas are among the most popular. You can make your own variations, using a ½ cup of fruit in combination with 4 tablespoons each of cachaça and sweetened condensed milk, a cup of ice, and a teaspoon of sweetener.

Coconut Batida
(Batida de Coco)

4 tablespoons *cachaça*
6 tablespoons coconut milk
4 tablespoons sweetened condensed milk
1 cup crushed ice
1 teaspoon Splenda
Sliced strawberries, for garnish

Place all ingredients in a blender and whip until smooth. Serve in a large martini glass garnished with sliced strawberries.

Servings: 1
Preparation time: 5 minutes or less

Peanut Butter Batida
(Batida de Amendoim)

4 tablespoons *cachaça*
3 tablespoons creamy natural peanut butter
4 tablespoons sweetened condensed milk
1 cup crushed ice
1 teaspoon Splenda
Pinch of chopped peanuts, for garnish
Pinch of stressed coconut, for garnish

Place all ingredients in a blender and whip until smooth. Serve in a small tumbler garnished with chopped peanuts and shredded coconut.

Servings: 1
Preparation time: 5 minutes or less

Strawberry Batida
(Batida de Morango)

4 tablespoons *cachaça*
½ cup fresh strawberries or thawed frozen strawberries
4 tablespoons sweetened condensed milk
Juice of ½ lime
1 cup crushed ice
1 teaspoon Splenda
Mint leaves, for garnish

Place all ingredients in a blender and whip until smooth. Serve in a tall glass garnished with mint leaves.

Servings: 1
Preparation time: 5 minutes or less

Limacello

I love the Italian liqueur limoncello. *It's an excellent aperitif for hot days, which are in ample supply in Brazil. To give it a Brazilian twist, I wanted to use the fragrant limes* (limas *or* limão *in Portuguese), which are so much a part of Brazilian cuisine, and* cachaça.

15 limes
4½ cups high-quality *cachaça*
5 cups water
4½ cups sugar

Wash and scrub the limes to remove all dirt and wax. Grate the zest from the limes. In a large jar, combine the zest and the *cachaça*. Seal tightly and place in a cool, dark place for two weeks.

After two weeks, retrieve the lime mixture. Using a sieve lined with muslin, cheesecloth, or filter paper, strain the mixture over a bowl. In saucepan over medium-low heat, dissolve the sugar in the water and keep it simmering for about 10 minutes. Remove from heat and stir the sugar syrup into the lime mixture. Use a funnel to pour the liquid into a 1-quart bottle, and seal. Store in a cool, dark place for a week, then chill in the freezer until ready to serve.

Servings: More than 30
Preparation time: 30 minutes to prepare, 3 weeks to mature

DRESSINGS, MARINADES, AND SAUCES

Garlic Wine Marinade
(Vinha d'Alho)

This foundation marinade, translated as "garlic wine," is the first step for virtually every Brazilian dish involving meat, poultry, or fish. The Portuguese brought to Brazil the tradition of marinading meats in their wines coupled with the indigenous spices found in the colonies they settled. The reach of this tradition extends beyond Brazil: in India, where the Portuguese had a stronghold on the western coast in such locales as Goa, vinha d'alho was not only the basis of the cuisine but also the name of dishes—hence the fiery curry known as vindaloo. The headiness of the garlic, the astringency of the wine and the limes, and the robust flavors of bay leaf and black pepper meld to produce an aroma and flavor that's uniquely Brazilian. In addition, preparing meats with this marinade provides such flavor to dishes that additional sauces can be superfluous, which helps to cut down on calories. Many combinations of this marinade exist; some cooks even guard their special formulas. After several trial-and-error attempts, I've come up with this particular recipe. Prepare a large batch of this marinade and keep it in a tightly sealed glass bottle in your fridge (it will keep fresh for about a week), so that you always have some on hand to make a quick meal.

4 cloves garlic, pressed
1 large onion, chopped finely
2 cups dry white wine (see Note)
Juice of 1 lime
3 tablespoons cracked black pepper
3 bay leaves
2 dashes of Tabasco or hot pepper sauce
1 teaspoon salt

Mix all of the ingredients, making sure to muddle the bay leaves carefully in the mixture to release their oils. Marinate red meats in a refrigerator for at least 3 hours; for

The Brazilian Bikini Body Program

chicken and pork, around 2 hours; for fish, no more than half an hour. When marinating steaks, pork, and poultry, be sure to really rub this mixture assertively into the meat with your hands.

Servings: More than 10
Preparation time: 5 minutes or less

Note: I love using Alsatian wines, Gewürztraminer, or Rieslings in this recipe for their sweetness, but good-quality Portuguese *vinho verde* also works well.

Green Aroma
(Cheiro Verde)

When traveling through Brazil's verdant expanse, you can't help but develop a sense memory of the powerful chlorophyll smell from trees and plants. Cheiro verde translates as "green aroma," due to its ingredients, and arouses a similar sensual experience. Like Garlic Wine Marinade this mixture features prominently in many dishes as a step in readying meat and vegetables, although it's less of a marinade and more of an herbal mélange. It's so versatile that you can adapt it for other uses. It makes a great sandwich topper, and works in a pinch as a salad dressing when mixed with a little olive oil and vinegar.

> 1 cup fresh curly-leaf parsley
> 1 cup fresh coriander
> 1 onion, chopped
> 1 scallion, chopped

With a mezzaluna or two knives, finely chop all the ingredients together until you have a uniform mixture. Keep in an airtight container in the refrigerator (it's usable for about four days).

Servings: More than 10
Preparation time: 5 minutes or less

Watercress Sauce
(Molho de Agrião)

Brazilians love their watercress, known as agrião. *It appears in salads, soups, stews, and even sauces, lending its characteristically peppery bite to every dish. This recipe makes a particularly nice foil for pasta, vegetables, steamed meats, and poached fish.*

> 2 tablespoons extra-virgin olive oil
> 3 cloves garlic, chopped finely
> 2 cups watercress
> 1 cup Green Aroma (page 77)
> Juice and zest of 1 lemon
> 1 teaspoon Tabasco or hot pepper sauce
> ¾ cup low-fat buttermilk or plain yogurt

Heat the oil in a large skillet and sauté the garlic until it softens.

As the garlic cooks, prepare a bamboo or metal steamer over a pot of boiling water. When the water is at a rolling boil, steam the watercress for about 30 seconds (keeping the lid over the steamer and pot), then remove the watercress and shock it in cold water. Drain and chop roughly.

Add the watercress, Green Aroma, lemon, and pepper sauce to the garlic, and cook until the mixture is uniform and heated through. Remove from heat and place in a blender. Add the buttermilk and puree until the sauce is smooth. Season with salt and pepper to taste.

Servings: More than 10
Preparation time: 5 minutes or less

Spinach Sauce
(À la Gula Gula)

My cousin Marcio and his partner Adriana introduced me to a chic and popular restaurant in Rio's trendy Leblon neighborhood called Gula Gula, which for the last two decades has spearheaded what the owners call Bossa Nova Cuisine. Vegetables and whole grains feature in the restaurant's menu of unusual salads, rich quiches, and grilled meats with sauces that don't trade flavor for healthiness. My favorite cold salad at Gula Gula consists of steamed broccoli, cauliflower, and mushrooms enrobed with a spinach sauce that resembles a green, vegetal aioli. This tasty sauce—which is essentially a basic mayonnaise flavored with spinach—pairs beautifully with salads, sandwich fillings, and cold meat spreads. I wanted to get a little additional sharpness and flavor into the mayonnaise, so here's my version of a spinach sauce similar to Gula Gula's.

1 cup fresh spinach (or thawed frozen spinach, squeezed of all moisture)

1 egg yolk

1 clove garlic, chopped

¼ teaspoon grated horseradish

1 teaspoon whole-grain mustard (Pommery is best)

1 cup extra-virgin olive oil

½ cup pickled capers

1 teaspoon lime juice

3 dashes of Tabasco or hot pepper sauce

4 tablespoons chicken or vegetable broth

Place the spinach in a steamer over a pot of boiling water and steam for 3 minutes. After 3 minutes, remove the spinach and shock it in cold water. Drain it and squeeze all the excess moisture out with your hands, then chop the spinach finely.

While the spinach steams, place the egg yolk, garlic, horseradish, and mustard in a blender or food processor, and beat slowly. Add the olive oil in a fine stream and continue beating until the mixture forms a mayonnaise and the oil is incorporated. Add the cooked spinach, capers, lime juice, pepper sauce, and broth, and continue beating for about 3 minutes, until everything is completely mixed. Add salt and pepper to taste. Serve cold.

Servings: 6
Preparation time: 10 minutes or less

Arugula Sauce
(Molho de Rucula)

Thanks to Brazil's large Italian immigrant history, gnocchi (spelled nhoque *in Brazil) can be found on menus everywhere. Although shoppers in the gorgeous daily markets of Rio and São Paulo can purchase the pillowy, potato-based pasta fresh, many prefer to make* nhoque *at home. Like pesto but tangier, this sauce is a classic mate for* nhoque; *it works equally well with roasted vegetables or slathered on good, fresh bread.*

> 2 cloves garlic
> 1 cup chopped arugula
> ¼ cup chopped fresh coriander
> ¼ cup walnuts
> ¼ cup cashews
> ¼ cup freshly grated Parmesan cheese
> ½ cup extra-virgin olive oil
> Juice of 1 lime

Wrap the two garlic cloves in foil and roast in a 375°F oven for 20 minutes, or until soft. Remove from foil. Place the garlic and all the other ingredients in a blender or food processer, and puree. Add salt and pepper to taste.

Servings: 8
Preparation time: 25 minutes or less

Chunky Vinaigrette
(Molho Vinaigrette/Molho Campana)

Brazilians are unabashed carnivores. The king-size barbecue houses known as churrascarias *are a riot of choice—for meats, for salads, and for the accompaniments that dress all that simply grilled flesh. My favorite of all the myriad Brazilian barbecue dressings is this salad-in-a-sauce. Mix its tart crunchiness into the steamed rice and roasted manioc flour usually served with grilled meat, and you have a classic Brazilian feast.*

3 tomatoes, chopped finely

2 onions, chopped finely

1 green bell pepper, chopped finely

1 clove garlic, pressed

3 tablespoons fresh parsley, finely chopped

2 tablespoons fresh coriander, finely chopped

½ teaspoon sugar or Splenda

1 cup organic apple cider or white wine vinegar

Mix all the ingredients together. Add salt and pepper to taste.

Servings: 8
Preparation time: 10 minutes or less

Nutty Mango Vinaigrette

Use this on salads. It can also be drizzled on fish and meat.

1 clove garlic, roasted

1 shallot, chopped finely

¼ cup chopped fresh coriander

¼ cup chopped fresh or thawed frozen mango

5 tablespoons rice vinegar

2 tablespoons mirin (Japanese cooking wine)

1 tablespoon ground cashews or Brazil nuts

2 tablespoons sesame oil

Place all the ingredients except the oil in a blender and puree until smooth. Pour the puree into a bowl and whisk the oil into the mixture. Add salt and pepper to taste.

Servings: 6
Preparation time: 10 minutes

Pepper Sauce
(Molho Apimentado)

This recipe really requires Brazilian-style preserved malagueta peppers. Substitutes just don't provide the same hot, vinegary flavor. You can buy jars of these peppers online (see Resources) and use them over a long period of time—they're so hot you'll use them sparingly, unless you actually enjoy sweating and crying simultaneously. Be careful: A little of this fiery sauce goes a long way, so adjust the use of the peppers to your liking. This is yet another great drizzling sauce for grilled, roasted, or poached fish. It does not keep well and is meant to be used only when fresh, so try to use it when you've got a lot of hungry people to feed.

3 malagueta peppers, mashed
½ teaspoon salt
1 onion, chopped finely
1 small unripe tomato, diced, or a tomatillo for even better flavor
1 teaspoon Green Aroma (page 77)
Juice of 1 lemon
Juice of 1 lime

Mash the first five ingredients together to form a paste. Then add the lemon and lime juices. Keep refrigerated in an airtight container.

Servings: 8
Preparation time: 5 minutes or less

Anchovy Sauce

The anchovy's briny, oily fishiness can be a big turnoff to uninitiated or finicky palates. But when drizzled sparingly over a grilled steak or poached white-fleshed fish, this sauce packs a bold punch that enlivens a simple preparation.

1 (2-ounce) can anchovy fillets in olive oil, drained
1 clove garlic, pressed
2 tablespoons finely chopped fresh parsley
2 tablespoons whole-grain mustard (Pommery is best)

3 tablespoons balsamic vinegar
½ teaspoon honey
½ cup extra-virgin olive oil

Place the anchovies, garlic, parsley, mustard, vinegar, and honey in a blender or food processor. Puree until smooth. Lower the setting so that the mixture beats slowly, and add the oil in a thin stream until it's incorporated. Add pepper to taste.

Servings: 8
Preparation time: 10 minutes or less

Pirão

Think of this protein-laden mush made with manioc flour as the Brazilian cousin of polenta. Like polenta, you can serve this in a "wet" form, or you can bake it into tasty croutons that lend crunch to salads or stand alone as a nutrient-rich starchy side dish.

1 pound fish heads (see Note)
1 onion, chopped finely
3 cloves garlic, pressed
1 cup Green Aroma (page 77)

¼ teaspoon salt
3 tablespoons extra-virgin
    olive oil
2 cups manioc flour

In a stockpot over medium heat, combine the fish heads, onions, garlic, and Green Aroma with 3 cups of water. Cook, uncovered, for 45 minutes, stirring occasionally, then strain the liquid and discard the solids. Add the salt and olive oil to the liquid, returning the pan to high heat. Add the manioc flour in small amounts, stirring constantly, until all the flour is added and the mixture has thickened.

Servings: 10
Preparation time: 1 hour

Note: You can ask your fishmonger for these scraps when you are buying fillets. They are usually happy to give you the scraps free of charge. Be sure they are from freshly filleted fish.

Acarajé Sauce

I love the savory bean fritters known as acarajé (page 100) so much, I've been known to wolf them down while they're still hot from the pan. But they truly get a lift when split open and served with this sauce. If you live in a big city, you might be able to find dendê oil and dried shrimp in African or Latin grocery stores. If these are not available, you can order both online (see Resources).

1 tablespoon grated fresh ginger
1 onion, chopped finely
2 tablespoons dried shrimp, soaked in water
2 mashed malagueta peppers or 1 teaspoon Tabasco
¼ cup Green Aroma (page 77)
3 tablespoons *dendê* oil

Place the ginger, onion, shrimp, peppers, and Green Aroma in a blender or food processor, and puree until smooth. In a skillet, heat the *dendê* oil and sauté the puree for 5 minutes. Add salt to taste.

Servings: 6
Preparation time: 15 minutes

Lime Sauce
(Molho de Limão)

This is the perfect quick sauce for fish. Cashews, a Brazilian staple, add a sweet nuttiness as well as a thickening agent to the sauce.

2 tablespoons extra-virgin olive oil
1 small onion, chopped finely
1 clove garlic, pressed
¼ cup ground cashews
Juice of 5 limes
1 small malagueta pepper, mashed, or 5 dashes Tabasco
 or hot pepper sauce

In a skillet, heat the oil. Add the onions and garlic, and cook until they soften. Add the cashews, mixing them into the onion mixture. Then add the lime juice and pepper, raising the heat and cooking until the sauce starts to bubble and thicken. Remove from heat. Use a food processor, blender, or hand blender to pulse the sauce until smooth. Add salt and pepper to taste.

Servings: 4
Preparation time: 10 minutes

Limacello Vinaigrette

Here's an easy recipe that makes use of the homemade lime liqueur that resembles a Brazilian version of Italy's limoncello. I was inspired by a limoncello vinaigrette recipe I tasted at Babbo, a New York Italian restaurant owned by the chef Mario Batali, and came up with my own version.

> ½ cup Limacello (page 75)
> Juice of 1 lime, with its zest
> 2 tablespoons whole-grain mustard (preferably
>   Pommery)
> ½ teaspoon Tabasco or hot pepper sauce
> ¼ cup extra-virgin olive oil

Whisk the liqueur, lime juice, zest, mustard, and pepper together until thoroughly mixed. Then add all the oil as you continue to whisk until smooth. Add salt and pepper to taste.

Servings: 6–8
Preparation time: 3 minutes

Coriander-Garlic Sauce

Nothing could be easier than this sauce. Its versatility is matched only by how quickly it can be prepared. Use it to marinate fish, poultry, and meat; add some apple cider vinegar to turn it into a salad dressing; spread it on bread for sandwiches; or drizzle on and mix it into hot pasta for a quick meal. If you have time, try to roast the garlic first before using it (you can do this by putting the cloves in their papery skins in a preheated 400°F oven for about 30 minutes, or until the garlic is soft).

1 cup fresh coriander, chopped finely
2 cloves garlic
½ cup extra-virgin olive oil
1 teaspoon black pepper
¼ teaspoon salt
½ teaspoon honey

Pulse all the ingredients to a smooth puree in a blender or food processor. Add salt and pepper to taste.

Servings: More than 10
Preparation time: 5 minutes or less

Shrimp Sauce
(Molho de Camarão)

Use this rich sauce to top grilled fish for a festive meal; to make a gratin with vegetables; or, if you're pressed for time, on its own with some whole grains and a salad. This recipe uses a mixture of buttermilk and reduced-fat sour cream, but if you're not watching your weight and you'd like to sample the traditional, Brazilian flavor of the dish, substitute ⅓ cup of cream instead.

2 tablespoons extra-virgin olive oil
1 clove garlic, minced
1 onion, chopped finely
½ pound shelled, raw shrimp, chopped
1 red bell pepper, seeded and chopped finely
1 tomato, chopped finely
¼ cup low-fat buttermilk
¼ cup reduced-fat sour cream
½ cup Green Aroma (page 77)
1 teaspoon salt
2 teaspoons cracked black pepper

Heat the oil in a skillet over high heat. Add the garlic and onions, stirring constantly as they turn golden. Add the shrimp and cook until they just start to turn pink. Remove the shrimp from the pan and set aside. Place the red pepper and tomato in the skillet, and add 1 more tablespoon of oil if needed. Cook until the mixture softens and thickens. Return the shrimp to the pan and add the buttermilk, sour cream, Green Aroma, salt, and pepper. Stir and let cook for about 1 minute, then serve immediately.

Servings: 4
Preparation time: 20 minutes or less

Gorgonzola Sauce
(Molho de Gorgonzola)

If you're cooking a very lean piece of red meat, such as buffalo, ostrich, or extra-lean beef, the lack of fat can yield the equivalent of a tasteless strap of leather. To keep things low in calories but high in flavor, sear and cook the meat no more than medium-rare; then dab it with a tablespoon or two of Gorgonzola sauce, which accentuates the meaty flavor. Gorgonzola sauce is a very popular accompaniment to meat in Brazil, thanks yet again to the Italian influence on the cuisine.

¼ cup low-fat buttermilk
¼ cup plain yogurt
¼ teaspoon Splenda
½ cup Gorgonzola, Roquefort, Stilton, or another high-quality blue
    cheese
2 tablespoons Green Aroma (page 77)

Place everything except the Green Aroma in a skillet over medium heat. Stir continuously until the mixture starts to bubble and thicken. Remove from the heat and whisk in the Green Aroma. Add cracked black pepper to taste.

Servings: 8
Preparation time: 10 minutes or less

SALADS

Lentil Salad
(Salada de Lentilhas)

Lentils are not only a nutritious, heart-healthy legume, they are also considered a symbol of good luck in Brazil. On New Year's Eve, one custom involves throwing lentils on the ground and stepping on them as midnight strikes. After the last bell tolls, many Brazilians serve and devour a version of this simple and tasty salad. For added fiber, you can throw in some baby spinach leaves or any salad greens you may have sitting around.

1½ cups Puy or small green lentils
1 tomato, chopped finely
1 onion, chopped finely
1 green bell pepper, seeded and chopped finely
1 red bell pepper, seeded and chopped finely
½ cup black olives, pitted and chopped finely

DRESSING
¼ cup red wine vinegar
4 tablespoons extra-virgin olive oil
2 tablespoons whole-grain mustard (preferably Pommery)
1 teaspoon tamari or soy sauce
½ teaspoon Splenda

Rinse the lentils, and cook until tender—about 20 minutes in boiling water. Drain the lentils and run them under cold water to cool. Mix with the chopped vegetables. In a separate bowl, whisk together the vinegar, oil, mustard, tamari, and sweetener into an emulsion, then pour directly over the salad. Toss the salad and serve cold.

Servings: 4
Preparation time: 20 minutes or less

Chickpea Salad
(Salada de Grão de Bico)

My mother is crazy about legumes. She loves having a lentil or chickpea salad available for snacking from the fridge at any time. The crunch and freshness of this salad makes it easy to pair with fish or lamb—or on its own as a filling, savory lunch, or snack. It actually tastes better on the second day, when the flavor of the bay leaf becomes more pronounced (just don't eat the bay leaf!). You can use the dressing below, or substitute ¼ cup of Limacello Vinaigrette (page 85).

2 cups cooked chickpeas (see Note)
1 bay leaf
1 red onion, chopped finely
3 stalks celery, chopped finely
1 green bell pepper, seeded and chopped finely
1 cucumber, peeled and chopped
1 cup cherry tomatoes, halved
¾ cup crumbled feta cheese
½ cup Green Aroma (page 77)

DRESSING
¼ cup red wine vinegar
4 tablespoons extra-virgin olive oil
¼ teaspoon honey or Splenda
1 teaspoon whole-grain mustard (preferably Pommery)
2 tablespoons cracked black pepper
Pinch of salt

Mix the beans, bay leaf, vegetables, cheese, and Green Aroma together in a bowl. In a separate bowl, whisk the vinegar, oil, sweetener, mustard, pepper, and salt into a dressing and pour over the salad. Toss the salad and serve cold.

Servings: 6–8
Preparation time: 10 minutes or less

Note: You can soak dried chickpeas overnight and cook them for 1 to 1½ hours, or use good-quality canned beans that have been rinsed and drained.

Black Bean Salad
(Salada de Feijão)

Black beans are the cornerstone of many Brazilian meals. Here they appear in a velvety and tangy cold dish that goes well with chicken, beef, or fish. As with the Chickpea Salad, you can use the suggested dressing or substitute ¼ cup of Limacello Vinaigrette (page 85).

2 cups cooked black beans (see Note)
½ cup Green Aroma (page 77)
1 onion, chopped finely
1 red bell pepper, seeded and chopped finely
1 yellow bell pepper, seeded and chopped finely
1 green bell pepper, seeded and chopped finely

DRESSING
¼ cup red wine vinegar
4 tablespoons extra-virgin olive oil
¼ teaspoon honey or Splenda
1 teaspoon whole-grain mustard (preferably Pommery)
2 tablespoons cracked black pepper
Pinch of salt

Mix the beans and vegetables together in a bowl. In a separate bowl, whisk the vinegar, oil, sweetener, mustard, pepper, and salt into a dressing and pour over the salad. Toss the salad and serve cold.

Servings: 4–6
Preparation time: 10 minutes or less

Note: You can soak dried black beans overnight and cook them for 1 hour, or use good-quality canned beans that have been rinsed and drained.

Broccoli and Cauliflower Salad
(In Homage to Gula Gula)

If you've got Spinach Sauce already prepared and sitting in the fridge, all you need to do is steam some vegetables, toss them with the sauce, and serve.

1 cup broccoli florets
1 cup cauliflower florets
1 cup shiitake mushrooms, sliced
½ cup Spinach Sauce (page 78)

Place the vegetables into a steamer and cook until al dente. Shock the vegetables in cold water to stop the cooking, and drain. Toss with Spinach Sauce and serve cold.

Servings: 4
Preparation time: 10 minutes or less (if Spinach Sauce is already prepared)

Classic Brazilian Salad

Every restaurant in Brazil offers this basic salad, usually as part of a set meal. The piquancy of the sliced radishes and the sweetness of the carrots provide the characteristic flavor. Use the suggested dressing, or try Nutty Mango Vinaigrette (page 81) as a substitute.

4 cups romaine lettuce, torn roughly into small pieces
1 cup radishes, sliced
2 carrots, julienned
2 tomatoes, sliced

DRESSING
¼ cup red wine vinegar
4 tablespoons extra-virgin olive oil
2 tablespoons cracked black pepper
1 dash of honey

Combine the lettuce, radishes, carrots, and tomatoes in a bowl. In a separate bowl, whisk the vinegar, oil, pepper, and honey into a dressing and pour over the salad. Toss the salad and serve cold.

Servings: 4
Preparation time: 10 minutes or less

Palm Heart Salad
(Salada de Palmito)

This is one of my all-time favorite salads. Palm hearts are delicate and nutty. Their sweetness perfectly balances the acidity of the tomatoes and the sharpness of the onion. I prefer this salad dressed with a vinaigrette made from Coriander-Garlic Sauce. But beware: After eating this much garlic and onion, make sure to have a mint on hand, or freshen your breath naturally by chewing on fresh parsley, ginger, or black licorice.

2 medium-size tomatoes, sliced
1 onion, sliced into rings
1 (14-ounce can) palm hearts, rinsed and sliced

DRESSING
4 tablespoons red wine vinegar
¼ cup Coriander-Garlic Sauce (page 86)

Lay the sliced tomatoes on a large plate. Layer them with the onion rings and then the sliced palm hearts. Whisk the vinegar through the Coriander-Garlic Sauce and drizzle over the vegetables.

Servings: 4
Preparation time: 10 minutes or less

Eggplant Salad
(Salada de Berinjela, Queijo, e Pirão)

Of all the food vendors plying their wares on Brazil's beaches, I find none more fascinating than the barbecued cheese man. Queijo coalho is a type of artisanal, firm-curd cheese made from raw milk, usually prepared by roasting over a charcoal grill. Beachside, vendors carry tiny portable hibachis which they use to barbecue skewers of these cheese cubes to order. This salad recipe was inspired by one that features queijo coalho, *taken from a 2002 cookbook called* Super Saladas. *If you can find curd cheese in your local shops, great! But if that proves too difficult, try this version, which substitutes the firm Greek cheese* halloumi, *and croutons made from* pirão. *To save on time, you can substitute precooked eggplant slices packed in olive oil, which are often sold at supermarkets or Italian specialty stores. If you're really pressed for time, leave out the croutons and substitute a handful of nuts (page 103). This hearty and substantial salad works well as a dinner entrée.*

2 tablespoons balsamic vinegar

4 tablespoons extra-virgin olive oil

Zest and juice of 1 lime

1 pound eggplants, cut into thick slices

½ cup Green Aroma (page 77)

1 cup Pirão (page 83)

½ pound *halloumi* or other curd cheese, cut into cubes

½ cup whole wheat flour

4 tablespoons cracked black pepper

1 head dark leaf lettuce

Pitted black gaeta olives

1½ cups cherry tomatoes

Make a dressing of the balsamic vinegar, 2 tablespoons of the oil, and the lime juice and zest. Preheat the oven to 350°F.

Stir the Green Aroma into the cold, leftover *pirão*, making sure to mix it thoroughly (moisten the leftover *pirão* with a little water, if required). Spread this mixture in a shallow baking dish that has been oiled with 1 tablespoon of extra-virgin olive oil. Bake at 350°F for 1 hour, or until the mixture has lost all its liquid and firmed up. Let the mixture cool completely. Turn on the oven broiler and prepare an oiled baking sheet.

While the *pirão* is cooling, dress the eggplant slices with a little bit of the rest of the olive oil, then steep each slice in the balsamic vinegar dressing. Place the slices on the cooking sheet, set under the broiler, and cook, turning them once, until both sides are soft and golden, approximately 8–10 minutes on each side. Remove from the heat.

While the eggplant is cooking, dredge the *halloumi* cubes in whole wheat flour and pepper.

Once the *pirão* has cooled, cut it into cubes. Arrange the *pirão* and *halloumi* cubes on the cooking sheet, moisten with some of the vinegar mixture, and place under the broiler for about 5 minutes, turning them lightly once, and roasting until the cubes and cheese turn golden brown. Remove from the heat.

Place lettuce, olives, and tomatoes in a salad bowl, adding the eggplant, cheese, and *pirão*. Dress with the rest of the vinegar mixture and the remainder of the olive oil.

Servings: 4
Preparation time: 1½ hours (includes crouton-baking time)

Watercress Salad
(Salada de Agrião)

Peppery and packed with iron and vitamin C, this basic salad serves as a great foil for red meat, but you can pair it with anything you like. It's delicious and good for you. If you're not keen on onions, sliced apples make a great substitute. The addition of hard-boiled egg adds some hearty protein to give the dish heft, and it's a common Brazilian touch in salads.

> 2 cups watercress, rinsed and chopped
> 2 palm heart stalks, chopped
> 1 onion, sliced, or 1 apple, cored and sliced
> 1 tomato, chopped finely
> 1 hard-boiled egg, chopped
> ¼ cup Limacello Vinaigrette (page 85), or other vinaigrette

Combine the vegetables and the egg in a large bowl. Toss with vinaigrette and serve.

Servings: 2
Preparation time: 5 minutes or less

Spinach Salad
(Salada de Espinafre)

Warm spinach salads beat cold ones by miles. The hot bacon will sufficiently heat the salad to wilt the spinach and warm the whole dish—allowing the flavors to meld and develop. This version substitutes turkey bacon for pork but, if you're not calorie-counting, use the real thing for that smoky flavor. There's just enough oil from the artichoke hearts to create a base for dressing the dish.

> 2 cups spinach, rinsed, well drained, and chopped
> ½ cup artichoke hearts in olive oil, drained and chopped
> ¼ cup cashews, chopped
> 2 tablespoons balsamic vinegar
> 1 tablespoon whole-grain mustard (preferably Pommery)
> 4 strips turkey bacon
> 2 tablespoons grated Parmesan cheese

In a large bowl, combine the spinach, artichoke hearts, and cashews. In a separate bowl, whisk together the vinegar and the mustard, and drizzle onto the salad. In a skillet, cook the bacon until golden. Then remove the bacon from the pan and, while still hot, add to the salad. Using a fork and knife, cut the bacon into the spinach and artichokes, making sure to integrate all the ingredients as you cut them into smaller pieces. Sprinkle with the cheese and serve.

Servings: 2
Preparation time: 20 minutes or less

Tuna Salad
(Salada de Atum)

Unlike heavy tuna salads swimming in mayonnaise, this one preserves the taste of the fish. A light dressing made with rice wine vinegar gives this salad a fresh accent. Use it as a sandwich filling, or accompanied with either mixed greens or shredded cabbage and carrots. One sandwich vendor on Ipanema beach makes this tuna as a filling for his "health-food sandwiches," making them unique among the heavy, waterlogged belly bombs you can get stuck with on the beach. Finding him on a busy, sunny day is like finding a needle in the haystack, so here's my approximation of the salad.

1 (6-ounce can) tuna in spring water, drained

1 red onion, diced

1 cucumber or pickle, peeled and diced

1 stalk celery, diced

4 tablespoons Green Aroma (page 77)

3 tablespoons rice wine vinegar

2 tablespoons extra-virgin olive oil

2 tablespoons lime juice

¼ teaspoon salt

1 teaspoon cracked black pepper

1 hard-boiled egg, chopped

In a large bowl, flake the tuna with a fork. Add the onion, cucumber, celery, and Green Aroma. In a separate bowl, whisk together the vinegar, oil, lime juice, salt, and pepper.

Pour the dressing onto the tuna salad and toss until thoroughly integrated. Sprinkle with the chopped egg.

Servings: 2–3
Preparation time: 10 minutes or less

SMALL BITES

Roasted Meatballs
(Quibe Assado)

The sizable immigrant communities from the Middle East brought this very popular dish to dining tables, snack shops, and restaurants all over Brazil. Called quibe *(kee-bee) in Portuguese, these meatballs are redolent with the aromas of allspice, mint, and nutmeg. Serve them along with some vegetables and a soup for a hearty meal, or grab one on the go for a satisfying protein pick-me-up.*

1 pound extra-lean lamb or
    ground beef
1 cup bulgur wheat, presoaked
    for about 20 minutes and
    completely drained
1 onion, chopped finely
¼ cup chopped mint leaves
1 tablespoon ground allspice

2 tablespoons ground cinnamon
1 teaspoon ground nutmeg
1 teaspoon ground cloves
½ teaspoon salt
1 teaspoon cracked black pepper
3 tablespoons extra-virgin olive
    oil

Preheat the oven to 375°F. In a large bowl, mix all the ingredients by hand to make sure they are well integrated. Rub your hands with a little bit of olive oil, and scoop a palm-size amount of the mixture, rolling it between your hands to make a small, stubby cigar shape. Continue to make patties out of the mixture in this way until none remains, and place the patties on a small rack over a shallow baking dish to allow the fat to drip down. If you don't have a rack, place the patties in the baking dish, oiled with the remainder of the olive oil, and be sure to drain the fat every 15 minutes from the pan while the patties are roasting. Roast the *quibe* for about 35 minutes—turning over the patties after about 15 minutes to cook evenly—or until browned and crispy.

Servings: 10
Preparation time: 45 minutes or less

Cheese Rolls
(Pão de Queijo)

No visitor to Brazil leaves without sampling the country's famous cheese rolls several times. Quite simply, when fresh out of the oven, these are among the tastiest cooked cheese delicacies in the world—able to hold their own against French gougères, Italian frico—and they definitely best anything cheesy-and-bready that comes out of American fast-food pizza chains. Puffy, airy, and tangy, cheese rolls' unique flavor is the result of the flour and the cheese: Fermented manioc starch (also known as tapioca flour) provides a zippy note that puckers the mouth; queijo de Minas (a regional, artisanal Brazilian cheese from Minas Gerais state) provides the salty gooeyness that never overwhelms and tastes just right. Many Brazilians make breakfast out of a large cheese roll and a tiny cup of inky espresso, but they also consider this a light snack. Serve these with a soup and salad for lunch or dinner. As a shortcut, I have been known to use packaged pão de queijo *mix (Yoki makes the best ones), adding freshly grated cheese to enhance the flavor. If you live in a big city with Brazilian grocery stores, you can easily find these mixes; otherwise, purchase the mixes online if you can't be bothered to attempt the recipe from scratch (see Resources).*

1 cup water
1 teaspoon salt
1 cup milk
2 cups tapioca flour
2 large eggs or 3 small ones
½ pound Gruyère or Parmesan cheese, grated (see Note)
½ cup extra-virgin olive oil

Preheat the oven to 350°F. In a saucepan over high heat, bring the water, salt, milk, and oil to a boil. Add the tapioca flour, and mix with a wooden spoon or spatula, taking care to smooth any lumps. Let the mixture cool. Put the mixture into a bowl, add the eggs, and knead the dough with your hands. Add the cheese and continue to knead until the dough is smooth and uniform. Rub your hands with a little bit of the olive oil, and scoop up a small amount of dough (about 1 heaping tablespoon), rolling it between your hands to make a Ping-Pong–size ball. Place all the balls on a greased cookie sheet and bake for approximately 20 minutes, until golden and crusty. Uncooked rolls can be frozen to be baked at a later time.

Servings: 20
Preparation time: 40 minutes

Note: If you live in a big city with good Brazilian or gourmet cheese shops, try to procure *queijo de Minas*.

Acarajé

Hands-down, acarajé are my favorite Brazilian treat. These crunchy, fluffy fritters made from black-eyed peas represent the best of Afro-Brazilian cuisine from Bahia—think of them as Brazilian-fusion falafel. Their unique flavor comes from dried shrimp and dendê palm oil, a viscous, bright orange vegetable oil. Restrict your use of this oil; it is a saturated fat and, while it does have some healthy properties, frying anything in it doesn't exactly do wonders for the waistline. That said, as occasional treats, acarajé are very well worth having. The acarajé's Bahian heritage means it should be spicy. But the heat factor can be dialed down by limiting how much hot sauce you use. Split the fritters in half and add a dollop of Acarajé Sauce (page 84) in the middle to make a little fritter-sandwich before devouring.

2 cups cooked black-eyed peas (see Note)
2 cloves garlic
1 onion, chopped finely
½ cup dried shrimp, soaked in water
1 tablespoon baking powder
1 teaspoon salt
1 tablespoon Tabasco or hot pepper sauce
½ cup canola oil
½ cup *dendê* palm oil

Make sure the peas and shrimp are well-drained; there should be no liquid in these ingredients when making the paste. Pulse the peas, garlic, onion, shrimp, baking powder, salt, and hot pepper sauce in a blender or food processor to form a coarse paste. Don't overprocess the mixture; it's okay if it's a bit lumpy. Wet your hands with a bit of water and scoop a small, palm-size amount of the paste into your hands to form a small patty. Continue making patties until all the paste is used; for best frying, you can refrigerate the patties for a half hour before frying them, but you can also fry them immediately. In a heavy-bottomed stockpot, heat the two oils together until shimmering. Slide small batches of the patties into the oil and fry until they are crisp and golden. Drain them on absorbent paper.

Servings: 10
Preparation time: 40 minutes

Note: You can soak dried black-eyed peas overnight and cook them for 1 hour, or use good-quality canned beans that have been rinsed and drained.

Salt Cod Fritters
(Bolinhos de Bacalhau)

Don't be daunted by this recipe. It features salt cod (or rather a salted substitute like scrod or pollock), which to some eyes (and noses) may appear as both unlovely and a lot of hassle. But while it requires a bit more effort than other recipes, the results are a tasty reward. Salt cod holds an extremely important gastronomic and historic place of pride in southern Europe and South America, where it is variously known as bacalhau *in Portuguese,* baccalà *in Italian,* bacalao *in Spanish, and* morue *in French. In Portugal especially, cod—the "beef of the sea"—is the cornerstone of the cuisine. When colonizers traveled to and settled in Brazil, the cod, salted and preserved for long voyages and storage times, came with them. This dish can be found in Europe as well as Brazil, where it appears as a snack, hors d'oeuvre, and first course. A few of them, along with a good salad, make for a terrific light dinner option.*

1 gallon milk
½ pound salt cod
2 bay leaves
10 peppercorns
1 onion, minced
1¼ cups mashed potatoes (see Note)
2 small eggs, beaten
¾ cup Green Aroma (page 77)
½ teaspoon Tabasco or hot pepper sauce
1 cup canola oil
Chopped parsley, for garnish

In the early evening of the day before you want to fry the fritters, place the salt cod with enough milk to cover it in a stockpot and soak it overnight. Change the milk in the pot before you go to sleep, and again in the morning. When you are ready to cook in the evening, take out the salt cod and rinse off the milk. Remove the skin and any bones, and cut the cod into small chunks. Rinse out the stockpot and place the cod chunks in it again with enough water to cover them. Add the bay leaves, peppercorns, and onion to the water. Bring the cod to a simmer, then turn off the heat and put a lid on the pot. If you don't have time to make the fritters now, you can store the cod in the refrigerator in this liquid until you're ready to use it.

To make the fritters, drain and flake the fish in a large bowl. Add the mashed potatoes and mix well. Add the beaten eggs, Green Aroma, and pepper sauce. Make sure all the ingredients are thoroughly incorporated into the mixture, then place the fish into the fridge for about a half hour to chill. Afterward, wet your hands with some water, and scoop a small, palm-size amount into your hands to form round balls. Fry in the canola oil in small batches and drain on absorbent paper. Serve with chopped parsley.

Servings: 10
Preparation time: 1 day for soaking, 1 hour to prepare and fry

Note: Use leftovers! To make fresh mashed potatoes, boil 3 large potatoes or 6 to 8 small ones in salted water until soft—approximately 40 minutes. Then mash the potatoes with ¼ cup of water or, if you prefer, skim milk.

Romeo and Juliet
(Romeu e Julieta)

This mild and creamy little snack is a sophisticated jolt of fruit and cheese. As the name implies, the combination seems unlikely at first, but the two flavors actually fit together beautifully. It's usually served as a dessert or cheese course, but if you keep the portion small— about the length of a stick of gum—it's an excellent tidbit to tide you over until your next full meal. Guava and quince pastes are available at Latin stores and major supermarkets.

½-ounce slice of guava or quince paste
½-ounce slice reduced-fat cream cheese

Layer the two slices together and enjoy.

Servings: 1
Preparation time: 5 minutes or less

Crunchy Nuts with Soy
(Castanhas Crocantes I)

Here's a tasty, healthy, and easy snack, featuring cashews, Brazil nuts, and pumpkin seeds—three highly nutritious ingredients that represent Brazil's bounty. Remember, these are tempting but rich. Take only one handful at a time! These are meant to be a snack to carry you over to your next meal.

> 1 cup cashews
> 1 cup Brazil nuts, chopped
> 1½ cups pumpkin seeds
> 2 tablespoons tamari or reduced-sodium soy sauce
> ½ teaspoon ground coriander
> ½ teaspoon garlic powder
> Pinch of cayenne

Preheat the oven to 350°F. Mix the tamari and spices together in a large bowl with the nuts, and toss. Spread out the nuts and seeds on a cookie sheet. Toast them in the oven until they turn golden and give off a nutty aroma—about 15 minutes—turning them midway.

Store in the freezer or in an airtight jar.

Servings: 15
Preparation time: 15 minutes

Crunchy Nuts with Chile and Lime
(Castanhas Crocantes II)

Adjust the amount of cayenne powder to your taste.

2 tablespoons lime juice
1 tablespoon balsamic vinegar
½ teaspoon garlic powder
½ teaspoon ground cumin
½ teaspoon cayenne
1 cup cashews
1 cup Brazil nuts, chopped
1½ cups pumpkin seeds

Preheat the oven to 350°F. Mix the lime juice, vinegar, and spices together in a large bowl, add the nuts, and toss. Spread out the nuts and seeds on a cookie sheet. Toast them in the oven until they turn golden and give off a nutty aroma—about 15 minutes—turning them midway.

Store in the freezer or in an airtight jar.

Servings: 15
Preparation time: 15 minutes

Honey-Nut Crumble
(Castanhas Crocantes III)

Use a handful of this nut crumble as a snack, or as a topping on desserts like Prune Compote (page 163) or Fruit Salad (page 162), or anything else you like.

2 tablespoons extra-virgin olive oil
1 teaspoon ground cinnamon
½ cup honey
1 teaspoon grated orange zest
1 cup cashews, chopped coarsely
1 cup Brazil nuts, chopped coarsely
1 cup shelled pumpkin seeds

Preheat the oven to 325°F. In a bowl, mix all the ingredients except the nuts and seeds. Then stir in the nuts and seeds, coating thoroughly. Spread the mixture onto an oiled cookie sheet and place in the oven. Bake for 20 minutes, or until the nuts and seeds caramelize, making sure to turn them over at the midway point. Remove from the oven when both sides are done and spread on a sheet of foil to cool. When completely cooled, crumble or break into pieces and store in an airtight jar.

Servings: 15
Preparation time: 20 minutes

SANDWICHES AND SOUPS

Brazilian Chicken Soup with Rice
(Canja de Galinha)

Every country has its variation on chicken soup, and Brazil is no different. Canja made an appearance in my family's house—as it would in most people's homes—whenever someone felt poorly (soup was usually followed by bananas sautéed with a touch of cinnamon sugar). It was also occasionally prepared after a roast chicken meal, as it uses up chicken leftovers quite nicely.

> 1 stewing chicken, cut into pieces
> 1 cup Garlic Wine Marinade (page 76)
> 3 tablespoons extra-virgin olive oil
> 3 cloves garlic, mashed
> 1 onion, chopped
> 1 bulb fennel, chopped
> 1 cup uncooked rice
> 2 bay leaves
> 1 teaspoon cinnamon
> 1 teaspoon cayenne
> 1 tomato, seeded and chopped
> 1 carrot, sliced
> 8½ cups water
> ½ cup dried porcini or shiitake mushrooms (optional)
> 1 cup Green Aroma (page 77)
> 1 cup spinach leaves (optional)

Marinate the chicken pieces in the Garlic Wine Marinade making sure to work the marinade into and under the skin of the chicken. Leave the chicken in the refrigerator for at least an hour, and preferably overnight.

In a large stockpot over high heat, heat the oil, then add the chicken, searing the chicken pieces until golden brown. Remove the chicken pieces and set aside. Add to the stockpot the garlic, onions, and fennel, sautéing until they soften. Add the rice, stirring rapidly to coat each grain with oil. Then add the bay leaves, cinnamon, cayenne, tomato, carrots, and finally the chicken. Add enough water to cover all the ingredients, lower the heat to medium, and place the lid on the pot.

Check the pot every 15 minutes for 1 hour, skimming the oily froth off the top. When the rice is cooked and the meat falling off the bone you may, if you wish, completely debone and remove the skin from the chicken and the soup. At this point, add the mushrooms if you have them.

Cook for another half hour, uncovered, to the point at which the liquid has reduced by half. Stir in the Green Aroma—and, if you wish, some fresh spinach leaves. Add salt and pepper to taste, and serve hot. Unused portions may be frozen.

Servings: 8
Preparation time: 2 hours (excluding marinating time)

Black Bean Soup
(Caldo de Feijão)

This soup might be the best way to introduce legumes to confirmed bean-haters. The smoky accent of the chouriço *marries perfectly with the hearty beans; the two together create a robust, meaty flavor that satisfies even the fussiest carnivores who claim to never touch legumes. This soup is quite rich and can be served as a meal on its own, especially if you chop up a few leaves of kale or spinach and toss them into the soup a few minutes before serving.*

> 2 cups cooked black beans (see Note)
> 2 cups chicken or vegetable broth
> ¼ pound *chouriço* sausage, chopped
> 4 cloves garlic, mashed
> 1 onion, chopped
> 1 bay leaf
> ½ teaspoon salt
> ¼ cup Green Aroma (page 77)

Place the beans and the broth into a food processor and puree until smooth. In a stockpot over medium heat, sauté the *chouriço* sausage until golden. Remove the sausage and reserve, and sauté the garlic and onions in the oil from the sausage. When browned, return the sausage to the stockpot and add the bean mixture, bay leaf, and salt. Place a lid on the stockpot and simmer the soup over low heat to allow the flavors to develop. After 10 minutes, taste and adjust the seasonings. Serve with the Green Aroma sprinkled on top of the soup.

Servings: 4
Preparation time: 20 minutes

Note: You can soak dried black beans overnight and cook them for 1 hour, or use good-quality canned beans that have been rinsed and drained.

Cream of Palm Heart Soup
(Sopa de Palmito)

I'll admit to having taken some license with this recipe. Palm heart soup is deliciously creamy and nutty when dairy is added sparingly. In the wrong proportions, the basic ingredients can result in an insipid and bland broth. To enliven the flavor and sharpen the taste of palm heart, I usually throw in a chipotle in adobo—admittedly a Mexican touch that would never appear in an authentic Brazilian kitchen. While Brazilians would use malagueta peppers, I prefer the heat and smoke of the chipotle, which rounds out the creaminess of the soup. You can find canned chipotles in adobo in many supermarkets, next to the salsas and taco shells. A warning: One chipotle gives quite a bit of heat. If you're not a spice enthusiast, cut the pepper in half and scrape out the seeds before adding to the dish. If you want to be indulgent, substitute ¾ cup of heavy cream for the buttermilk and sour cream.

3 tablespoons extra-virgin olive oil or 1 tablespoon butter
1 onion, chopped finely
1 (14-ounce) can palm hearts, sliced
2 cups chicken stock
½ cup buttermilk
¼ cup reduced-fat sour cream
1 chipotle in adobo
¼ cup Green Aroma (page 77)

In a stockpot, heat the oil or melt the butter over medium heat and sauté the onions until they are about to turn golden. Add the remaining ingredients and bring the soup to a boil. Reduce the heat, partly cover the pot, and simmer the soup for 5 minutes. Remove it from the heat and place into a food processor. Puree the soup until smooth and then return it to the pan. Bring the soup to a boil over low heat and stir frequently for approximately 3 minutes.

Servings: 6
Preparation time: 15 minutes

Caldo Verde

This soup originally hails from Portugal, where common staples like chouriço *sausage and kale feature prominently in the cuisine. When Portuguese colonizers came to Brazil, their cuisine became one indelible part of Brazil's gastronomic spectrum. Caldo verde (which translates as "green broth") is a potage much like the French vichyssoise, but more nutritious given the addition of kale. The vegetable's color not only gives the dish its name, it also serves as the cook's alert. Kale is the last thing added to the soup and it should only be cooked for a few minutes— to the point at which it turns a brilliant emerald color. When you see that vivid green, take the soup off the heat immediately and serve, otherwise the kale will overcook and turn a dull brown.*

> ¼ cup extra-virgin olive oil
> 2 cloves garlic, mashed
> 1 onion, chopped finely
> 1 pound small potatoes, cleaned and sliced (see Note)
> 8 cups water
> ¾ pound *chouriço* or smoked sausage, sliced thinly
> 1 pound kale, washed thoroughly and cut into fine shreds
> Splash of olive oil

In a stockpot, sauté the garlic and onion in the oil over high heat. When the onions soften, add the raw potatoes, stirring constantly to coat each slice with oil, for approximately 2 minutes. Add the water, place the lid on the pot, and bring to a boil over medium heat. Cook for 15 minutes, or until the potatoes are soft. If you are using already cooked leftover potatoes, add the water, and cook the potatoes for only about 30 seconds before taking them out of the water. Do not discard the cooking liquid.

While the potatoes cook, fry the sausage in a skillet until golden. Drain the sausage slices on absorbent paper and set aside.

Remove the potatoes from the water, place them in a food processor, and puree, adding 2 cups of the reserved cooking water. Return the potato puree to the stockpot water, along with the sausage, and salt and pepper to taste. Replace the lid and simmer over medium heat for 5 minutes. When ready to serve, stir the kale into the potato broth and simmer, uncovered, for about 3 minutes, or until the kale turns bright green. Add a splash of olive oil on top before ladling into serving bowls.

Servings: 6
Preparation time: 40 minutes or less

Note: Yukon Gold or fingerling potatoes work best; you may also use leftover cooked potatoes.

Watercress Soup
(Sopa de Agrião)

Brazilians rarely have to worry about cold weather. On hot days, Brazilians prize their watercress's crunchy coolness. But when living in cities like London, Paris, New York, or Amsterdam (all of which have large and vibrant Brazilian communities), they turn the peppery leaf into a rich, warming soup for wintry days. If you're watching calories, substitute buttermilk for the cream.

1 teaspoon butter
1 clove garlic, chopped
1 onion, chopped
¼ cup Green Aroma (page 77)
2 cups chicken broth
1 pound watercress, rinsed and chopped
1 cup milk
¼ cup heavy cream or low-fat buttermilk

In a stockpot over medium heat, sweat the garlic and onion in the butter until they soften. Add the Green Aroma, stirring rapidly until the leaves start to wilt. Add the chicken broth, and turn the heat up to high. When the broth starts to come to a boil, add the watercress and turn the heat down, bringing the liquid to a simmer. Cook the watercress for about 2 minutes, then add the milk and remove the mixture from the heat. Pour into a food processor or blender. Pulse until the mixture is smooth and uniformly green. Pour the soup back into the stockpot over low heat, cover the pot, and simmer for another 15 minutes to allow the flavors to develop. Stir in the cream, heat for another minute, then serve.

Servings: 6
Preparation time: 30 minutes or less

Miso Soup

In Liberdade, the Tokyo-esque district of São Paulo, some people eat a cheese roll and coffee for their breakfast, some guzzle down a fruit smoothie, but quite a few more reach for a small pot of miso soup. The significant and unique diaspora of Japanese to Brazil has made its stamp on the national cuisine. In São Paulo, where the Japanese influence is strongest and most visible, even the humblest restaurants may offer miso soup, yakisoba, kaki-age, or yakitori on the menu. But whether in Tokyo or São Paulo, most families save time when making something as basic as miso soup by using hon-dashi powder (also called dashi-no-moto) as a shortcut. Making miso soup from scratch requires boiling a large strip of kelp and katsuo-bushi (dried bonito tuna flakes), a somewhat wasteful and time-consuming practice. Hon-dashi eliminates those steps by freeze-drying and granulating the kelp and fish into a dissolvable powder. With it, preparing miso soup takes only a few minutes and thus can be had in a snap as a starter to your lunch or dinner. For a nutritious start to the day, you may do as many do and enjoy it as a quick and wholesome breakfast.

4 cups water
2 teaspoons *hon-dashi* powder
1 block firm fresh tofu, cut into cubes
5 shiitake mushrooms, sliced
4 tablespoons red miso
1 scallion, sliced

In a stockpot over high heat, boil the water, then add the *hon-dashi*. Stir and dissolve the powder completely. Add the tofu and mushrooms, lowering the heat to simmer gently for 2 minutes. Add the miso and stir until fully dissolved. Turn off the heat, add the scallion, and serve.

Servings: 4
Preparation time: 10 minutes or less

Bauru Sandwich

São Paulo is the birthplace of Brazil's most famous sandwich, named after the residential neighborhood of its creator. In a still-standing, eighty-year-old bar called the Ponto Chic, a student named Casimiro Pinto Neto layered roast beef, melted cheese, tomatoes, and pickles on a crusty French bread loaf and gave birth to a standard that remains one of Brazil's most popular lunch choices.

> 1 small whole wheat French bread roll
> 2 slices tomato
> ¼ teaspoon dried or fresh oregano
> 6 pickle slices
> 1 slice Emmentaler or Swiss cheese (regular or reduced-fat)
> 2 thinly cut medium-size slices of roast beef or cooked leftover steak

Turn on a broiler to preheat it. Toast the roll lightly and slice it lengthwise. Rub the tomato slices into one half of the roll. Sprinkle the oregano over the tomato and add a layer of pickles, then cheese. Place this half under the broiler to melt the cheese for about 1 minute. Layer the steak over the melted cheese, add salt and pepper to taste, press the other half of the roll onto the sandwich, and serve hot.

Servings: 1
Preparation time: 5 minutes or less

Natural Sandwich
(Sanduiche Natural)

In Brazil, what passes for natural or its loose translation, "health food," would shock a lot of granola-munchers (although, that said, granola can contain alarmingly high doses of sugar and fat, making it far from healthy as well). On the beach, sandwich vendors hawk lots of types of sanduiches naturais, but most feature mayonnaise; limp, wilted fillings of iceberg lettuce; and a few sad shreds of carrot. Every now and then, a beach-goer can get lucky and find a good sandwich-maker. I did when I stumbled on a mobbed vendor whose customers were grabbing her offerings, bursting with fresh, crunchy shredded vegetables. I've replicated an approximation of that tasty filling here, and encased it in a wrap for easier portability. This sandwich is a great way to use up leftover salad leaves before they go bad; add leftover tomatoes, sliced hard-boiled eggs, tofu, or any other favorite nonmeat ingredients lurking in the fridge to add heft and avoid food going to waste.

½ cup shredded arugula
1 tablespoon chopped beets
1 small carrot, shredded
½ red bell pepper, seeded and sliced
3 cashews, chopped finely
4 walnut halves, chopped finely
1 tablespoon lime juice
1 tablespoon tamari or reduced-sodium soy sauce
1 teaspoon grated fresh ginger
½ teaspoon extra-virgin olive oil
3 drops sesame oil
2 slices whole wheat bread or 1 small whole wheat wrap

Mix in a bowl all the ingredients except the bread. Place between bread slices or roll into the wrap, and serve.

Servings: 2
Preparation time: 5 minutes

Falafel

As they have to so many countries around the world, immigrants from places like Syria and Lebanon brought the delightfully crunchy and filling falafel fritter to Brazil. Falafel, esfihas (a cheese and meat turnover pastry), quibe (page 98), and hummus are so popular that a Middle Eastern fast-food chain called Habib's has grown nationwide to become one of Brazil's largest restaurant franchises. Try this Lebanese falafel recipe, which uses equal amounts of chickpeas and fava beans, giving the inside of the fritter a lovely green color.

1 cup chickpeas, soaked overnight (see Note)
1 cup fava beans, soaked overnight (see Note)
1 clove garlic, chopped
1 red onion, chopped
½ cup Green Aroma (page 77)
1 teaspoon baking powder
1 teaspoon salt
½ teaspoon ground cumin
1 teaspoon Tabasco or hot pepper sauce
½ cup canola oil

FALAFEL YOGURT SAUCE
2 tablespoons plain yogurt
1 tablespoon Green Aroma (page 77)
½ teaspoon Tabasco or hot pepper sauce
Pinch of salt and pepper

Put the chickpeas and favas into a food processor. Add the garlic, onion, Green Aroma, baking powder, salt, cumin, and hot pepper sauce. Make a coarse paste by pulsing the mixture, scraping down the sides of the processor after approximately every five pulses. Add a few tablespoons of water to loosen the mixture and continue to process until green and uniform (a few small lumps are okay; just be sure not to overprocess the mixture into a mush). Place the paste in a bowl.

Heat the oil in a heavy-bottomed skillet until it shimmers. With either your hands (wet them with water first) or two tablespoons, scoop and shape the falafel mixture into small, rounded patties. Slide them carefully into the hot oil and fry in small batches until crisp and brown. Drain on absorbent paper.

Mix together all the yogurt sauce ingredients and drizzle onto the hot falafel.

Servings: 6
Preparation time: 30 minutes

Note: You can use dried legumes, or substitute good-quality canned chickpeas and fava beans. Be sure to drain and rinse the beans before use. (Please be aware that fava beans can be fatal to some people.)

MEAT

Churrasco

Churrasco means "barbecue," and in Brazil, barbecue means "carnivorous orgy." Visitors to Brazilian rodizio steakhouses understand this after gorging themselves on the seemingly endless parade of grilled meats served by waiters from sword-like spits. In much the same way that American barbecue aficionados proudly trumpet their smoking and saucing techniques from region to region, Brazilians are no less fanatical. The Brazilian barbecue difference is in minimalism, emphasizing the cut of the meat rather than a sauce. Brazilians also prefer beef to pork, with the only basting coming from salmoura, a solution of coarse sea salt in water brushed onto the meat, using a mop of coriander. The salt water creates a crusty, char-grilled exterior to the meat that seals in its juiciness. As in most parts of the world, the combo of meat and fire brings out primal competitiveness in men, and my father and cousins Roger and Marcio will forever vie for the title of churrasco king. This recipe features their very simple technique. Serve the meat with Chunky Vinaigrette (page 80).

> ½ cup coarse sea salt
> 1 cup water
> 1 bunch fresh coriander
> 1 pound beef tenderloin, cut into 4 thin, even pieces (ask your
>   butcher to do this)
> 4 well-marbled steaks

In a bowl, preferably wooden, mix the water and the salt to make the *salmoura*. Tie the coriander at the stems with a twist-tie or clip, to make a brush. Dip the coriander brush into the *salmoura* and baste the meat with it. When the grill is white-hot, place the meat over the center of the heat. Baste on both sides with *salmoura*, using the coriander brush every few minutes. When all the meat is brushed, shake off any excess salt, let it rest for a few minutes, then slice and serve.

Servings: 8
Preparation time: 30 minutes

Roast Pork Loin
(Lombo de Porco Assado)

Brazilians crave red meat, but special occasions often feature a lombinho or "little pork loin." Lean pork loin serves as a culinary blank canvas on which spices and sauces can stand out. Marinated first, then roasted, pork loin should be sliced thinly when served. Leftovers make excellent sandwich meat, so be sure to save some for the next day. For an extra kick, follow the recipe and spread a layer of whole-grain mustard over the whole loin before covering in foil and roasting. The juices in the roasting pan can be reduced to make a sauce for the loin: After removing the loin, place the pan on a stovetop burner and deglaze it by adding a cup of dry white wine (or, if you haven't got any at hand, a little extra Garlic Wine Marinade). Scrape all the brown bits into the liquid, then add a tablespoon of mustard, and a tablespoon of whole wheat flour or cornstarch. When thickened, add salt, pepper, and a touch of honey to taste, and pour over the tenderloin slices.

> 2-pound pork loin, as lean as you can find
> 1 cup Garlic Wine Marinade (page 76)
> 2 tablespoons coarse salt
> 2 tablespoons extra-virgin olive oil

Rub the pork loin with the salt. With a knife, score small cuts into the loin before placing it into a shallow casserole dish. Pour the Garlic Wine Marinade over the loin and work the marinade into the meat. Cover and place in a refrigerator to marinate for at least 2 hours, but preferably overnight. Make sure to turn the loin at least once so that the marinade penetrates all of the meat.

Preheat the oven to 325°F. Rub the pork with olive oil before placing it in the oven, and cover the top of the loin with foil. Roast the loin for about 1 hour, turning it on the half hour to ensure even cooking. Then remove the foil cover, raise the heat to 350°F, and roast for another half hour, or until the loin's surface is crisp and juices run clear when a knife is inserted. Keep a close eye on the meat during the last half hour to avoid overcooking and toughening it.

Servings: 8
Preparation time: 1½ hours (not including marinating time)

Brazilian Stroganoff

How did a French dish made by the cook of a Russian diplomat in the late 1800s become such a Brazilian favorite? Partly because of the Francophilic streak that runs through Brazilian cuisine, but mostly because of the large number of European immigrants who brought the recipe with them when they settled in Brazil during the nineteenth and twentieth centuries. Yet again, the dish's popularity serves as an indication of just how Brazilian food constitutes one of the world's most literal melting pots. The creamy Stroganoff sauce works with either beef or chicken and tastes best when served over rice—a Brazilian twist on the recipe's original accompaniment of egg noodles. If you want to add a real Brazilian (but indulgent and fatty) flair, sprinkle a few matchstick fried potatoes over the Stroganoff. You don't have to use cream; the substitute mixture of buttermilk and reduced-fat sour cream tastes equally rich but contains less fat.

> 2 pounds lean beef fillet or boneless chicken breast, cut into small
>   strips
> 1 cup Garlic Wine Marinade (page 76)
> 3 tablespoons olive oil
> 2 cloves garlic, minced
> 1 medium-size onion, chopped finely
> ½ cup chopped shiitake mushrooms
> ½ teaspoon salt
> ½ teaspoon ground nutmeg
> 1 teaspoon dried oregano
> ½ cup heavy cream, or ½ cup buttermilk and ½ cup reduced-fat sour
>   cream
> 4 tablespoons ketchup
> 3 tablespoons whole-grain mustard (preferably Pommery)
> 1 tablespoon Worcestershire sauce

Marinate the meat for at least 1 hour (or preferably overnight) in the Garlic Wine Marinade, in the refrigerator.

In a large skillet, heat the oil over medium heat. Add the garlic and onion, and cook until they just start to soften. Raise the heat to high and add the meat, searing it until browned. Add the mushrooms, salt, nutmeg, and oregano, combining the ingredients thoroughly in the pan. Add some of the Garlic Wine Marinade and turn the heat to low. Cook for about 10 minutes, or until the mushrooms have released their liquid and gone soft. Then add the ketchup, mustard, and Worcestershire sauce and stir. After the mixture starts to bubble slightly, add the cream and cook for 1 more minute, stirring to combine thoroughly. Adjust the seasoning with black pepper. Serve over rice or with a salad.

Servings: 6
Preparation time: 30 minutes (not including marinating time)

Brazilian Mincemeat
(Picadinho)

Mincemeat usually finds its way into patties of some kind, but try using it plain or as a vegetable stuffing the way Brazilians do. My version of picadinho incorporates the traditional salty chopped olives and diced peppers, as well as a Japanese-based seasoning that brings out the flavor of both the meat and the vegetables. I recommend this recipe for any ground meat— not just beef. It works superbly with ground turkey, which also reduces the total amount of fat. Use it as a stuffing for hollowed-out zucchini, squashes, pumpkins, or bell peppers (roasting the stuffed vegetables under medium heat for 20 minutes before serving), or serve plain with rice and vegetables.

> 2 strips turkey bacon
> 1 tablespoon olive oil
> 1 clove garlic
> 2 onions, chopped
> 2 malagueta peppers, minced, or 1 teaspoon Tabasco or hot pepper
>   sauce
> 1 green bell pepper, seeded and chopped
> 1 pound extra-lean rump steak, chopped, or extra-lean ground beef or
>   ground turkey
> 2 tablespoons Worcestershire sauce
> 1 tablespoon tamari or soy sauce
> 2 tablespoons mirin (Japanese rice wine)
> 2 tablespoons tomato paste
> 2 bay leaves
> 3 tomatoes, chopped
> 1 cup pimiento-stuffed green olives, chopped
> 1 hard-boiled egg, chopped finely

In a large skillet, cook the bacon over high heat. When the bacon crisps, lower the heat, remove the bacon and drain it on absorbent paper, and set aside, keeping the fat in the pan. Add the olive oil to the fat and sauté the garlic, onions, malaguetas, and green pepper over low-medium heat. While they cook, whisk together in a bowl the Worcestershire sauce, tamari, mirin, and the tomato paste into an emulsion and set aside. When the vegetable mixture has softened, add the meat and turn the heat back to high. Once the meat has browned, add the emulsion, the bay leaves, tomatoes, and olives, stir thoroughly, and lower the heat to medium so the mixture can stew down, cooking for approximately 10 minutes. Stir occasionally, taste, and adjust seasonings. Remove the bay leaves and crumble the bacon into the mixture, sprinkling the top with the chopped egg before serving.

Servings: 4
Preparation time: 30 minutes or less

Wagoner's Rice
(Arroz de Carreteiro)

On the arid plains of southern Brazil's vast ranches, gauchos often must remain far from a warm kitchen while they tend to grazing herds. But being Brazilian, they insist on good food featuring their toothsome and well-flavored beef. So campfire-fueled one-pot stews reign in Brazil's cattle country. To make a filling and nutritious meal, this hearty pilaf requires nothing more than a simple green salad to accompany it.

2 pounds beef, cut into cubes
1 cup Garlic Wine Marinade (page 76)
1 tablespoon coarse salt
3 tablespoons freshly cracked black pepper
2 cloves garlic, chopped
1 cup Green Aroma (page 77)
4 tablespoons extra-virgin olive oil
1½ cups uncooked rice
1 large onion, chopped

2 tomatoes, seeded and chopped
1 red bell pepper, seeded and chopped
1 yellow bell pepper, seeded and chopped

Place the beef cubes into a large bowl and pour the Garlic Wine Marinade over it. Mix thoroughly and refrigerate for an hour, or overnight if you wish.

In a mortar or large bowl, mash together the salt, pepper, garlic, and half the Green Aroma to form a paste. Heat the oil in a large stockpot; when it starts to shimmer, add the meat, searing it so that the cubes brown on all sides. Do this in batches, so as not to crowd the meat and stew it. When all the meat is browned and set aside in a separate bowl, add a little of the Garlic Wine from the marinade to deglaze the pot, making sure to scrape all the brown bits into the liquid. Add the green paste, stirring rapidly to integrate the paste into the oil and wine. Add the rice and stir rapidly to coat each grain with the mixture, then add the onion, tomatoes, and peppers, followed by the beef, stirring thoroughly each time a new ingredient is introduced.

Pour enough water into the pot to cover all the ingredients, and bring to a boil. Cover the pot, reduce the heat, and simmer for about 25 minutes, or until all the water has been absorbed and the rice is cooked. Before serving, stir the rest of the Green Aroma into the rice, reserving a little to sprinkle on top as a garnish.

Servings: 8
Preparation time: 40 minutes (not including marinating time)

Cozido

Italians—a nationality which constitutes an enormous faction of Brazil's now-integrated immigrant community—will recognize this dish as bollito misto (translated from the Italian as "mixed boil"; in Portuguese, cozido simply means "cooked"). While this used to be a way to tenderize old and tough meats and vegetables, cozidos can certainly feature meats and vegetables of good quality now. After being cooked, the ingredients can be served hot or cold, and the spiced water they simmer in becomes a hot broth. The platter's various meats and vegetables can be packed for picnics, or sliced and layered into sandwiches. Make sure to have your favorite sauces on hand to serve with the cozido.

1 pound lean flank steak, quartered

1 cup Garlic Wine Marinade (page 76)

4 *chouriço* sausages

2 bay leaves

1 large sprig curly-leaf parsley

2 tablespoons black peppercorns

4 cloves garlic, sliced

4 whole cloves

1 small cabbage, cored and cut into wedges

2 ears corn on the cob, halved

1 carrot, cut into chunks

1 sweet potato, quartered

4 small new potatoes, halved

1 hard-boiled egg, sliced

DRESSINGS

Watercress Sauce (page 78)

Spinach Sauce (page 78)

Chunky Vinaigrette (page 80)

The night before you prepare this recipe, marinate the steak in the Garlic Wine Marinade, in the refrigerator.

When you're ready to prepare the meal, place the steak and sausages in a large pot, and add enough water to cover. Bring the water to a boil, skimming the froth off the top. Then add the bay leaves, parsley, peppercorns, garlic, and cloves. Reduce the heat to medium, cover the pot, and simmer for about an hour; the sausages should be removed after about a half hour, when they are cooked through. Set them aside, keeping them warm. When the steak is done, remove it and keep it with the sausages.

Skim all the froth off the top of the cooking liquid, then add the vegetables and a bit more water if necessary to cover them completely. Check the pot after about 15 to 20 minutes and remove the vegetables when they are tender. If some vegetables are cooked through sooner than others, take them out and reserve with the meat.

When all the ingredients have been removed from the broth water, arrange the meat, vegetables, and egg slices on a decorative platter. Serve with Watercress Sauce, Spinach Sauce, or Chunky Vinaigrette. Strain the cooking liquid and serve as a broth; the broth can also be frozen for use at a later date.

Servings: 4–6

Preparation time: 2 hours or less (not including marinating time)

Black Bean and Meat Stew
(Feijoada)

A separate book would be required just to cover the gastronomic, social, historical, and political implications of feijoada, *Brazil's national dish. At first glance, it's a stew of meat and black beans. But delve a little deeper by talking to Brazilians and you begin to uncover the regional importance of different preparations. The complexity and variety of accompaniments can set off passionate debate: They may include everything from sliced oranges, fried banana croquettes, and sautéed kale to fried manioc flour—all served with fluffy rice. One thing can never be in doubt: Feijoada is a rich meal that should be eaten earlier in the day to allow for complete digestion. This Rio-style recipe is typically served in restaurants for Sunday lunch, thereby allowing stuffed diners a chance to wallow lazily in the sun on the beach for the rest of the afternoon.*

Plan a brunch party around it, as this stew's serving portions were made for convivial and large gatherings. Remember to serve this with Chunky Vinaigrette (page 80), Pepper Sauce (page 82), Kale, Minas Style (page 146), and Rice with Broccoli (page 149). A caipirinha or batida (pages 69 and 73, respectively) go quite well with this meal!

> 1 pound lean beef chuck
> 1 pound pork shoulder
> 1 cup Garlic Wine Marinade (page 76)
> 1 pound lean bacon, chopped
> 2 cloves garlic, minced
> 2 medium-size onions, minced
> 1 pound smoked pork shoulder
> 1 pound *chouriço* sausages
> 4 cups dried black beans, soaked overnight and drained (see Note)
> 1 stalk celery, minced
> 4 bay leaves
> ½ cup chopped fresh parsley
> 1 teaspoon dried thyme
> 1 tablespoon salt
> Freshly ground black pepper
> 3½ quarts water

The night before you prepare this recipe, marinate the beef and pork shoulder in the Garlic Wine Marinade in the refrigerator. Then when you're ready to prepare the meal, brown the bacon with the garlic and onions in a large, heavy-bottomed stockpot over medium heat. When they start to turn golden, add all of the other ingredients and bring the mixture to a boil. Reduce the heat to low, cover the pot, and simmer the stew for about 2 hours.

After 2 hours, skim any froth off the top of the stew and test the meats. Remove each piece of meat once it is fork-tender. When all the meat has been removed, allow the beans to continue cooking for another half hour, or to the point that the liquid turns creamy and thick. Slice the meats and arrange on a platter. Serve the beans in a crock or large tureen, and arrange dishes with the various sauces and accompaniments around the platter and tureen.

Servings: 10
Preparation time: 3 hours or less (not including marinating time)

Note: You can substitute canned black beans, but this is one recipe where the dried beans make the difference.

Beef with Onions
(Bife Acebolado)

Beef and onions, what could be simpler? Grill some lean beef, caramelize sliced onions with a touch of balsamic vinegar, and serve both with a salad for a meal that requires less than 20 minutes to prepare.

> 4 lean beef fillets
> 1 cup Garlic Wine Marinade (page 76)
> 2 large onions, sliced into rings
> 3 tablespoons balsamic vinegar
> 3 tablespoons extra-virgin olive oil
> Cracked black pepper

The night before you prepare this recipe, marinate the beef in the Garlic Wine Marinade, in the refrigerator.

When you're ready to prepare the meal, toss the onion rings with the balsamic vinegar in a large bowl. Heat half of the olive oil in a skillet and sauté the onions over high heat until soft and caramelized. Set aside the onions and keep them warm. Brush the rest of the oil onto the steaks, season with the pepper, then sauté or grill them to the desired level of doneness. Arrange the meat on a serving platter and smother with the onions.

Servings: 4
Preparation time: 20 minutes (not including marinating time)

Grilled Beef with Sauce
(Bife Grelhado com Molho)

The sauce is the star of this recipe, so choose your favorite. Use a pastry brush to "paint" the steak with the sauce, ensuring that you add flavor but not too many calories to what should be a light dish.

> 4 lean beef fillets
> 1 cup Garlic Wine Marinade (page 76)
> 1 tablespoon olive oil
> Cracked black pepper
> 4 tablespoons sauce of your choice (see Note)

The night before you prepare this recipe, marinate the beef in the Garlic Wine Marinade, in the refrigerator.

When you're ready to prepare the meal, brush the beef with the olive oil, add the pepper, then grill the beef to the desired level of doneness. With a pastry brush, glaze the fillets with the sauce of choice and serve.

Servings: 4
Preparation time: 20 minutes (not including marinating time)

Note: Use Gorgonzola, page 88; Anchovy, page 82; Chunky Vinaigrette, page 80; Watercress, page 78; or Spinach Sauce, page 78.

Oxtail and Watercress Stew
(Rabada)

Oxtail may appear crude or unappealing to those who turn their nose up at offal. But that's only because they haven't eaten it in the right preparation. Slow-cooked in wine, the oxtail meat melts off the bone, and the bite of the watercress offers a sharp counterpoint to the beef's richness. As with other Brazilian one-pot meals, you can begin preparing this early in the day and let it sit cooking for hours while you go off to do other things. Just check regularly to make sure enough liquid remains in the pot during the cooking process.

> 2 pounds oxtails, cleaned, cut, and trimmed of almost all fat (ask your
>   butcher to do this)
> 2 cups Garlic Wine Marinade (page 76)
> 4 strips bacon, chopped
> 1 teaspoon butter
> 3 cloves garlic, minced
> 1 large onion, chopped
> 1 teaspoon salt
> 2 tablespoons freshly ground pepper
> ½ cup whole wheat flour
> 3 tablespoons tomato paste
> 2 cups high-quality beef stock
> 2 cups red wine
> 3 bay leaves
> 1 pound watercress, chopped
> ½ cup Green Aroma (page 77)

The night before you prepare this recipe, marinate the oxtails in the Garlic Wine Marinade, in the refrigerator.

When you're ready to prepare the meal, fry the bacon in a large stockpot until it starts to crisp. Remove the bacon and drain on absorbent paper. Add the butter, garlic, and onions to the bacon fat and cook until they soften. Remove the garlic and onion once they start to turn slightly golden. Roll the oxtails in salt, pepper, then the flour, and add them to the pot to sear over high heat for approximately 5 minutes. Do this in batches so that the oxtails are not crowded in the pan.

While the oxtails are cooking, whisk in a bowl the tomato paste into the beef stock, until completely dissolved. When all the oxtails have been browned, place them in the pot and add the bacon, garlic, onions, wine, bay leaves, and the beef stock mixture. Replace the lid, and lower the heat. Simmer the oxtail stew for around 3 hours, checking every half hour to make sure enough liquid is covering the oxtails, and to skim the fat and froth off the top of the liquid. If necessary, add a bit more water, broth, or wine to cover. After 3 hours, taste and adjust the seasonings, then stir in the watercress and Green Aroma. Cook for another 5 minutes, and serve.

Servings: 4
Preparation time: 3½ hours (not including marinating time)

SEAFOOD

Stuffed Crab Shells
(Casquinha de Siri)

Special dinner parties at my parents' house usually featured this decorative first course. As soon as I saw my mother rummaging through the kitchen cabinets to find the right tableware, I eagerly anticipated this creamy, crunchy gratin. Among all the delicious recipes my mother might occasionally prepare, by far this was my favorite. Typically, this dish is cooked and served in the crab's carapace (casquinha de siri means "crab's little shell"). My mother favored delicate scallop shells, which you can find in gourmet stores. However, shallow ramekins or ovenproof saucers work equally well.

2 small onions, chopped finely

1 tomato, seeded and chopped finely

½ red bell pepper, seeded and chopped finely

¼ cup Green Aroma (page 77)

3 tablespoons extra-virgin olive oil

1 bay leaf

½ pound lump crab meat

Juice of 2 limes

¼ teaspoon cayenne

1 tablespoon whole wheat flour

1 egg, beaten

½ cup grated Parmesan cheese

¼ cup panko bread crumbs

6 empty crab shells or ramekins

In a food processor or blender, pulse together the onions, tomatoes, pepper, and Green Aroma. Heat the oil in a lidded saucepan and add the mixture from the food processor, along with the bay leaf. Stir, then cover and cook over medium heat for about 3 minutes.

Turn on the oven broiler. Add the crab meat, lime juice, and cayenne, and some salt and pepper to taste, to the saucepan. Replace the lid and cook over low heat for about 10 minutes. Add the flour and the beaten egg to the crab meat mixture and stir rapidly to combine, until it thickens and the egg is slightly cooked. Spoon the mixture into crab shells. Combine the cheese and panko crumbs, then sprinkle over the crab mixture. Broil until bubbling and golden, about 3 minutes. Serve garnished with some Green Aroma sprinkled on top.

Servings: 6
Preparation time: 30 minutes or less

Vatapá

The best seafood dishes from Brazil generally come from Bahia, the coastal port region whose importance in Brazil's slave trade left a unique gastronomic legacy: African cuisine fused with Brazil's indigenous and colonial influences. Bahia's position on the Atlantic, with its bounty of fish, crab, and shrimp, meant that seafood played a central role in meals. Vatapá, an African seafood stew based around white-fleshed fish, also uses ground nuts as a thickener. Pair this with rice or serve with some steamed broccoli for a substantial meal.

½ cup dried shrimp

2 tablespoons grated fresh ginger

2 preserved malagueta peppers, mashed, or 2 fresh red chiles, seeded and chopped, or 2 tablespoons Tabasco or hot pepper sauce

2 tablespoons *dendê* oil

2 cloves garlic, mashed

1 large onion, chopped

2 cups fish or shrimp stock, or 4 cups chicken stock

1 cup coconut milk

Juice of 1 lime

1 pound white-fleshed fish fillets, such as gray sole, hoki, or halibut, sliced

1 pound shrimp, peeled and deveined

½ cup ground cashews

½ cup ground peanuts

½ cup bread crumbs

½ cup Green Aroma (page 77)

Salt and freshly ground black pepper

Soak the dried shrimp in warm water to cover for 15 minutes. Drain, then puree in a blender or food processor with the ginger and peppers. Set aside.

Heat the *dendê* oil in a large stockpot over medium-high heat. Sauté the garlic and onions until soft. Add the dried shrimp mixture and cook for 3 minutes. Add the stock, coconut milk, and lime juice, and cook until reduced by half, about 10 minutes. Reduce the heat to medium. Add the fish and simmer until almost cooked through, about 5 minutes or less. Then add the shrimp and simmer until pink and cooked through. Add the nuts, bread crumbs, and Green Aroma, stirring rapidly to combine and thicken the mixture to a paste-like consistency, cooking for another 3 minutes. Season to taste with salt and freshly ground black pepper.

Servings: 6–8
Preparation time: 40 minutes or less

Moqueca

Moqueca is an all-purpose term that implies stewing seafood in coconut milk. Moquecas can be made with fish, crab, lobster, and more; here I include the perennial Brazilian favorite of shrimp moqueca. Bahian dishes like this involve spicy peppers, but you can adjust the heat to suit your taste. Season with the pepper sauce drop by drop, sampling as you proceed.

2 tablespoons extra-virgin olive oil
6 cloves garlic, chopped finely
1 large onion, chopped
2 bay leaves
2 large tomatoes, seeded and chopped
Juice of 2 limes
1 (14-ounce) can coconut milk
3 tablespoons ground cashews
2 tablespoons malagueta pepper sauce or Tabasco or hot pepper sauce
1 pound shrimp, peeled and deveined
½ cup fresh coriander, chopped finely
3 tablespoons *dendê* oil

Heat half the olive oil in a stockpot until shimmering. Add half of the chopped garlic and chopped onions, and sauté until golden. Then add the bay leaves, tomatoes, and half of the lime juice, stirring thoroughly as the mixture cooks down and starts to thicken. After about 5 minutes, add the coconut milk, cashew nuts, and pepper sauce, stirring the sauce until it starts to bubble—about 1 minute.

While the vegetables are cooking, heat the other half of the oil in a skillet over high heat. Sauté the rest of garlic and onions until soft, then add the shrimp and cook until they start to turn pink. When the shrimp are barely cooked through, add the rest of the lime juice and stir, scraping down the sides of the pan. Then transfer the shrimp and lime juice to the stockpot, adding the coriander. Stir to mix the *moqueca*, and continue to heat for another minute or two. Drizzle the *dendê* oil on top and serve hot with rice.

Servings: 6
Preparation time: 30 minutes or less

Simple Roasted Fish
(Peixe Assado)

Roasting a whole fish is quick and easy. Don't be intimidated. Just ask your fishmonger to scale, gut, and clean the fish completely. All you need to do is season it and pop it into the oven. Make sure the fish is as fresh as possible. It should not have a fishy smell; the flesh should spring back to the touch; and the eyes should be bulbous, clear, and bright. If you're squeamish about the eyes and head of the fish, simply lop off the head with a sharp cleaver and freeze it so that you can boil it for fish stock at another time.

> 1 whole roasting fish, such as sea bass or snapper
> 1 lemon
> 4 tablespoons olive oil
> 1 clove garlic, minced
> 1 bay leaf
> 1 tablespoon freshly ground black pepper
> Lemon and lime wedges, for garnish

Preheat the oven to 350°F. Rinse the fish and pat dry thoroughly, including inside the cavity. Squeeze the juice of the lemon on the fish both inside and out, and rub lightly with your fingers. Then rub the fish with the oil inside and out. Chop the squeezed lemon rind into pieces and insert into the fish cavity, along with the garlic, bay leaf, and pepper. Place the fish on a lightly oiled roasting pan and insert into the oven. Roast for around 20 minutes for medium-size fish (estimate around 10 minutes for each inch of thickness of the fish). Serve garnished with lemon and lime wedges.

Servings: 4–6
Preparation time: 30 minutes or less

Simple Fried Fish
(Peixe Frito)

The star of many beachside Brazilian restaurant meals, fried fish should be greaseless, crunchy, and hot. Serve the fish immediately once it's been drained on absorbent paper, with sauce of your choice, such as Watercress Sauce (page 78) or Chunky Vinaigrette (page 80).

   ½ cup whole wheat flour
   3 tablespoons freshly ground pepper
   4 white-fleshed fish fillets, such as hoki, gray sole, halibut, or plaice
   4 tablespoons canola oil or other light oil
   2 to 3 sprigs curly-leaf parsley

Mix the pepper into the flour. Dredge the fillets in the flour. Heat the oil in a skillet until it shimmers. Cook the fish until golden on both sides, and drain on absorbent paper. Garnish with parsley and serve.

Servings: 4
Preparation time: 15 minutes or less

Cashew-Crusted Baked Fish
with Lime Sauce
(Peixe com Nozes a Molho de Limão)

Marinating the fish will slightly "cook" it, so the time in the oven is very short—just enough to crisp the nutty coating. You can use any remaining ground nuts to thicken the sauce.

> 4 white-fleshed fish fillets, such as hoki, gray sole, or plaice
> ½ cup Garlic Wine Marinade (page 76)
> ½ cup finely ground cashews
> 2 tablespoons extra-virgin olive oil
> ½ cup Lime Sauce (page 84)

Preheat the oven broiler. Marinate the fish in the Garlic Wine Marinade for 10 minutes, in the refrigerator.

Spread the ground cashews in a thin layer over a plate. Remove the fish fillets from the marinade and dredge them in the ground cashews, carefully pressing the nuts into both sides of the fish. Oil a cookie sheet with the olive oil and place the fish on top. Put the fish under the broiler and cook for 2 minutes or so, until the nut crust turns golden. Flip the fish over and cook the other side until done. Be careful to keep a close eye on the broiler to prevent the fish from overcooking. The fish should be completely cooked in about 5 minutes or less. Serve with the Lime Sauce drizzled over the fish.

Servings: 4
Preparation time: 20 minutes or less

Shrimp and Egg Bake
(Tortinha de Camarão)

When I'm exhausted after work and need to make something simple, I often turn to this recipe. Like making an omelet, you use up eggs in the fridge and cook everything in one skillet. To further save on time, I use frozen peeled shrimp straight from the freezer. A heavy-bottomed skillet is essential, something preferably cast iron. Don't use pans with plastic handles, or they'll melt in the oven!

3 tablespoons extra-virgin olive oil

1 clove garlic, minced

½ onion, chopped

½ green bell pepper, seeded and chopped

½ tomato, seeded and chopped

3 palm hearts, sliced

¼ pound shrimp, peeled and deveined

1 tablespoon Tabasco or hot pepper sauce

¼ cup chopped fresh coriander

½ teaspoon salt

1 tablespoon freshly ground pepper

4 eggs, beaten

Preheat the oven broiler to 400°F. Heat the oil in a cast-iron or heavy-bottomed skillet over high heat and sauté the garlic, onion, and peppers for about 2 minutes. Add the tomato and palm hearts, and let cook for about 2 minutes more.

Add the shrimp and stir the mixture rapidly, cooking until the shrimp just begin to turn pink. While the shrimp cooks, in a bowl add the hot pepper sauce, coriander, salt, and pepper to the beaten eggs, whisking rapidly to incorporate all the ingredients. Once the shrimp starts turning pink, drain any excess liquid, then pour the beaten eggs into the skillet and let the *tortinha* cook until the edges set—about 2 minutes. Place the skillet in the oven under the broiler and cook the egg mixture for another 2 minutes, or until the *tortinha* starts to turn golden on top. Remove it from the oven, let it set for about 30 seconds, then slide the *tortinha* onto a serving plate. Cut into slices and serve.

Servings: 4
Preparation time: 15 minutes or less

Cod Gomes de Sá
(Bacalhau a Gomes de Sá)

Salt cod makes another appearance in this roasted dish. Gomes de Sá was a Portuguese cod merchant from Porto who lived during the nineteenth century and who, according to legend, created the recipes for this famous dish as well as Salt Cod Fritters (page 101). This very Portuguese combo of cod and olives can be quite salty, but the potatoes and egg balance out the salinity. Drizzle olive oil over the dish before serving. You can serve it immediately after cooking or place this in the refrigerator overnight to be served the following day, to allow the flavors to develop.

½ pound new potatoes (Yukon Gold or fingerling are best), sliced thinly
½ pound salt cod, soaked in milk overnight and drained, or use fresh firm white fish like Pacific cod
¼ cup extra-virgin olive oil
1 clove garlic, sliced
1 large onion, sliced
½ cup pitted black gaeta olives
¼ cup chopped parsley
2 hard-boiled eggs, sliced

Preheat the oven to 375°F. In a stockpot of boiling water, cook the potatoes until tender, approximately 10 minutes. While the potatoes cook, remove the skin from the cod and flake the fish with your hands to remove any bones. Cook the cod in boiling water in a lidded stockpot over high heat for 5 minutes. While the cod cooks, heat half the oil in a skillet over high heat, and cook the garlic and onions until they soften, about 3 minutes. Place the rest of the oil in a roasting pan and add the cooked potatoes, cooked cod, and the garlic and onions. Toss the ingredients and place the pan in the oven. Roast for 15 minutes, or until the cod and potatoes start to brown. Remove the pan from the oven and arrange the mixture on a serving platter. Toss with the parsley and olives. Layer the slices of egg on top before serving.

Servings: 3–4
Preparation time: 40 minutes

Nigiri Sushi and Sashimi

Brazilians will look for any excuse to congregate and party, especially if food is involved. But if you can't be bothered to make feijoada *for a group of your friends and family, consider a sushi party instead. The key is finding sashimi-grade fish—and an extremely sharp knife to slice thin, even pieces. Once you've cooked the rice, all you need to do is set the table with a pot of the rice; a plate with squares of pre-cut nori; dishes of wasabi and pickled ginger; small dipping plates of soy sauce for each guest; and a platter with the sliced fish. Guests simply take a square of seaweed in hand and put a spoonful of rice in the center. Follow with a dab of wasabi on the rice and top with a piece of fish. Roll up the seaweed and eat. The sushi and sashimi can be accompanied with Hijiki Salad (page 152) or a green salad, if you wish.*

> 1 cup uncooked Japanese short-grain rice
> ½ teaspoon salt
> 1 tablespoon sugar
> 3 tablespoons rice wine vinegar
> ½ pound sashimi-grade raw tuna or a variety of other raw fish, such
>   as salmon, mackerel, or yellowtail
> Sheets of roasted nori, hand-cut size
> Tamari
> Pickled ginger
> Wasabi paste

Prepare the rice by rinsing it until the water runs clear. Cook according to package directions until done and let the rice rest for 10 minutes. Dissolve the salt and sugar in the vinegar. Fluff the rice, then add the vinegar mixture to the rice, combining thoroughly. Slice the fish into thin pieces with a very sharp knife. Arrange a platter with the sliced fish, sheets of nori, tamari for dipping, ginger, and wasabi. Place the rice into a covered bowl and serve along with the platter.

Servings: 2
Preparation time: 30 minutes or less

POULTRY

Brazilian Chicken Pot Pie
(Empadas de Galinha)

Brazil's concept of fast food has so many more variants than the usual burger-and-pizza joints that clot our public spaces (and arteries). One of my favorites is a chain of pie-shop franchises called Casa da Empada ("Home of Pies"), where they make delicious mini pies with fillings ranging from the Anglophilic cheese-and-onion; to a Japanese soy-marinated pork; to a ragu of palm hearts; to broccoli and cheese; to shrimp with spicy tomato sauce; to a classic Brazilian-style chicken pot pie. Empadinhas (translated as "little pies," the diminutive of empada) *have traditionally been served as snacks or* hors d'oeuvres. *But when filled with such tasty and wholesome ingredients, they can be paired with a salad to make a great lunch or light dinner. This recipe is also the basic recipe for the* empada, *which is simply a larger, casserole-size version of the pie. The bigger pie was a staple in my parents' home as a Sunday brunch/lunch/all-day meal, served with a salad and picked at throughout the course of a lazy weekend. Brazilians would wag their finger at me for not endorsing the idea of making the piecrust from scratch; however, when pressed for time, you need to employ a little* jeitinho *and take shortcuts. I prefer Pillsbury's ready-made frozen piecrusts, as they are close in flavor to the crumbly, friable pastry that distinguishes Brazilian pot pies.*

2 9-inch round frozen piecrusts, defrosted

3 tablespoons extra-virgin olive oil

1 large onion, chopped finely

1 clove garlic, chopped

2 boneless chicken breasts, chopped into cubes or strips, or leftover
    cooked chicken (preferable and tastier)

1 large tomato, chopped

2 bay leaves

½ cup pimiento-stuffed green olives, chopped

¾ cup palm hearts, chopped

1 teaspoon Tabasco or hot pepper sauce

Preheat the oven to 375°F.

Empadinhas
(Mini-Pies)

Take a rolling pin and roll out half the dough so that it is approximately ⅛ inch thick. Cut eight approximately 6-inch circles by pressing a small bowl into the dough. Oil an eight-muffin tin with a tablespoon of the olive oil and place one circle in each indentation. Roll out the other half of the dough, as before, cutting out another eight circles to reserve for the pie tops.

Empada
(Large Pie)

With half of the dough, line a casserole dish that has been oiled with 2 tablespoons of the extra-virgin olive oil. Make sure to smooth out bumps and gaps in the pastry. Reserve the other half for the pie top.

Filling

In a skillet, heat the remaining olive oil and add the onions and garlic, sautéing until golden. Raise the heat to high and add the chicken, browning the meat on all sides. When the chicken is cooked on the outside, add the tomato and bay leaves, cooking until the chicken mixture starts to thicken and stew down, about 2 minutes. Then add the olives, palm hearts, and pepper sauce, stirring rapidly to combine all ingredients thoroughly. Taste for seasoning and add salt, pepper, and perhaps a bit of sweetener (Splenda, a splash of balsamic vinegar, or a squeeze of honey) to taste. Remove the bay leaves and turn off the heat.

If making an *empada*, fill the pastry-lined casserole dish with the chicken mixture. Drape the pie top over the mixture and roll the sides of the piecrust over the top crust to seal the pie, trimming off any additional crust before sealing. Prick the top of the empada with a fork and place into the oven.

If making *empadinhas*, place 2 heaping tablespoons of the filling into each pastry-lined muffin cup. Drape each reserved pie top over a filled cup, carefully folding over the sides of each crust around the top to form a seal. With a fork, prick each pie on top to allow steam to escape and place the muffin tin into the oven.

Cook for 25 minutes, or until the piecrusts turn golden. The *empada* can be served directly from the casserole dish. To remove the mini-pies from the tin, slide a knife around the edges of each pie after they've cooled and gently upend the tin so that the pies can tumble out. Uneaten pies can be frozen for later use.

Shrimp Pies

Substitute 1½ pounds of small shrimp for the chicken and add ¼ cup of Green Aroma along with the palm hearts and olives.

Ground Beef Pies

Substitute 1 pound of ground beef for the chicken and add ¼ cup of Green Aroma along with the palm hearts and olives.

Palm Heart Pies

Substitute 2 (14-ounce) cans of chopped palm hearts for the chicken. Sauté the palm hearts with all other ingredients until fully cooked and well mixed.

Servings: 4–6 (*empada*) or 8 (*empadinhas*)
Preparation time: 1 hour

Ximxim de Galinha

The Bahian origin of this chicken stew is reflected in the use of such African staples as dried shrimp, ground nuts, peppers, and dendê oil. Even its name has an African origin. As with any Bahian dish, take care to adjust the seasoning to suit your taste, since this dish can be fiery.

2 whole chicken breasts, cut into strips
1 cup Garlic Wine Marinade (page 76)
4 tablespoons extra-virgin olive oil
3 cloves garlic, minced
2 onions, chopped
1 large tomato, chopped
1 red bell pepper, seeded and chopped

Juice of 3 limes
2 bay leaves
1 cup Green Aroma (page 77)
¼ cup chopped mint leaves
2 tablespoons grated fresh ginger
2 tablespoons *dendê* oil
½ cup ground cashews
½ cup ground peanuts
¼ cup ground dried shrimp

In a large bowl, pour the Garlic Wine Marinade over the chicken. Allow the chicken to marinate in the refrigerator for at least an hour, and preferably overnight.

In a large skillet, heat half the oil until it shimmers. Sear the chicken until golden on all sides, then remove from the pan and set aside. Add the other half of the oil to the pan over high heat and sauté the garlic and onions for 2 minutes. Then add the tomatoes, pepper, lime juice, bay leaves, Green Aroma, mint, and ginger, and cook for 3 minutes as it stews down. Then add the chicken, salt and pepper to taste, and 4 tablespoons of water. Reduce the heat to medium and cook the mixture for 20 minutes, adding a little water every 5 minutes when necessary. When the chicken is completely cooked, add the *dendê* oil, cashews, peanuts, and dried shrimp. Cook for another 5 minutes, then serve garnished with some Green Aroma sprinkled on top.

Servings: 4–6
Preparation time: 40 minutes

Garlic Chicken
(Frango à Passarinho)

This chicken recipe resembles both French and Asian preparations that feature a bird smothered in copious amounts of garlic. The Brazilian version undergoes two cooking processes: roasting and frying. This crisps the chicken and seals in juiciness. The fried garlic adds more crunch, as well as its delicious, distinctive flavor. On the whole, this dish makes a tasty alternative to heavy, breaded fried chicken.

> 1 chicken, cut into pieces, skin removed
> ½ cup Garlic Wine Marinade (page 76)
> 5 tablespoons canola or other light oil
> 1 head of garlic, chopped (about 15 cloves), or 10 tablespoons
>   prepared chopped garlic

Preheat the oven to 375°F. In a shallow baking dish, marinate the chicken pieces in the Garlic Wine Marinade for 30 minutes, in the refrigerator. Then place the chicken in the oven to roast for 20 minutes, turning over the pieces after 10 minutes. Remove the chicken pieces from the oven, drain on absorbent paper, and set aside.

In a large, heavy-bottomed skillet over high heat, fry the garlic in the oil until golden, then remove. Fry the roasted chicken pieces in the same oil until they are crispy and golden. Arrange the chicken pieces on a platter and smother with the fried garlic.

Servings: 4–6
Preparation time: 30 minutes (not including marinating time)

Roast Chicken
(Galinha Assada)

A juicy, crisp roast chicken is one of life's great gifts. Learning how to roast a chicken isn't difficult; just marinate first and baste regularly. Regulate the temperature, too: If you don't cover the chicken breast for the main part of the cooking period, it will dry out.

1 roasting chicken
1 cup Garlic Wine Marinade (page 76)
2 tablespoons extra-virgin olive oil
3 tablespoons freshly ground black pepper
2 tablespoons coarse sea salt
1 pound assorted root vegetables, including potatoes, parsnips, and
    sweet potatoes, cut into chunks

In a deep bowl, marinate the chicken in the Garlic Wine Marinade, making sure to rub it into and under the skin (separate the skin from the meat with your fingers), then place it in the refrigerator for 30 minutes.

Preheat the oven to 375°F. Remove the chicken from the refrigerator, and rub the olive oil into and under the chicken skin. Then rub the salt and pepper into the chicken.

Lay the root vegetables at the bottom of an oiled roasting pan and set the chicken on top of the vegetables. Cover the chicken breast with foil and place the roasting pan in the oven. Roast for 30 minutes, basting the meat every 15 minutes. After 30 minutes, remove the foil and roast for another 20 minutes, or until the skin is golden and crisp, and the juice runs clear when the leg is pricked with a knife. Serve the roast on a platter with the roasted vegetables arranged around it.

Servings: 4–6
Preparation time: 1 hour (not including marinating time)

Grilled Chicken
(Galinha Grelhada)

When firing up the barbecue grill, consider this marinade for making simple but savory chicken breasts. Don't worry if you don't have a grill; you can also cook the chicken in this fashion under a broiler.

> 2 whole chicken breasts
> ½ cup Garlic Wine Marinade (page 76)
> 4 tablespoons olive oil
> 4 tablespoons Coriander-Garlic Sauce (page 86)

Cut the breasts into four pieces and marinate in the Garlic Wine Marinade for 30 minutes, in the refrigerator. Heat and oil a grill with the olive oil. Brush the chicken breasts with the Coriander-Garlic Sauce and grill, turning every few minutes to cook evenly. Serve the chicken with more Coriander-Garlic Sauce.

Servings: 4
Preparation time: 20 minutes (not including marinating time)

Sautéed Turkey Breast
(Peitinho de Peru)

Thin turkey cutlets, a Brazilian lunch favorite, make this a quick meal to cook. Serve these with a salad and vegetables, and you have yet another meal in less than half an hour. Serve with Spinach Sauce (page 78) or Chunky Vinaigrette (page 80).

> 1 whole turkey breast
> ½ cup Garlic Wine Marinade (page 76)
> 2 tablespoons extra-virgin olive oil
> 1 clove garlic, minced

Cut the turkey breast into four pieces. Place the pieces between two sheets of plastic wrap, one at a time, and pound the breasts until thin and almost translucent. If possible, marinate the turkey breast in the Garlic Wine Marinade for at least half an hour before cooking.

Heat the oil in a skillet and sauté the garlic until golden. Remove the garlic from the pan, drain on absorbent paper, and set aside. Then add the turkey fillets to the oil and cook until seared on both sides. Arrange the turkey on a platter and scatter the garlic over the meat.

Servings: 4
Preparation time: 15 minutes (not including marinating time)

VEGETABLES

Efó

Slaves from West Africa brought not only their food and cooking techniques to Brazil, but also their languages. In a few West African dialects, efó means "greens," which are the focus of this Bahian spinach and shrimp dish. The presence of Bahian flavors predominate: smoky dried shrimp, coconut milk, nuts, and dendê oil. It can be served as a side dish, but it's substantial enough to star as the entrée when paired with rice.

2 tablespoons dried smoked shrimp

1 pound cooked shrimp, peeled

2 cloves garlic, minced

2 large onions, quartered

2 preserved malagueta peppers, mashed, or 2 tablespoons Tabasco
    or hot pepper sauce

3 tablespoons minced fresh coriander

3 pounds fresh spinach, washed thoroughly, stems removed, and
    shredded

2 tablespoons olive oil

2 large ripe tomatoes, chopped coarsely

Salt and freshly ground black pepper

1 (14-ounce) can coconut milk

½ cup ground peanuts

½ cup ground cashews

2 tablespoons *dendê* oil

Combine the smoked and cooked shrimp, garlic, onions, peppers, and coriander in a food processor or blender, and pulse the mixture to a coarse paste. Place the spinach in a colander in a large, covered saucepan and steam for 5 minutes over boiling water. Set the spinach aside. In a medium-size, heavy skillet, heat the olive oil over medium heat. Add the shrimp paste and cook, stirring a few times, until golden. Discard the water from the spinach-steaming saucepan and return the pan to medium heat, adding the shrimp mixture, spinach, tomatoes, and salt and pepper to taste. Stir in the coconut milk, peanuts, cashews, and *dendê* oil. Stir rapidly as it cooks for 5 minutes. Check the seasoning before serving.

Servings: 4
Preparation time: 25 minutes or less

Kale, Minas Style
(Couve à Mineira)

The key to Brazilian kale dishes is in the preparation of the vegetable. Brazilians eat kale finely shredded, cut into a "chiffonade": Roll the rinsed leaves into a tight cylinder. Then slice the cylinder in very thin slices, making fine ribbons of the leaves.

> 2 tablespoons extra-virgin olive oil
> 2 cloves garlic
> 4 strips peppered bacon, or 1 small dried *chouriço* sausage, chopped
> finely (optional)
> 4 cups finely shredded kale, washed and dried

Heat the oil in a skillet until shimmering. Add the garlic and if desired, the bacon or sausage. Cook until golden, then add the kale, stirring rapidly as the leaves cook down. Add salt and pepper to taste.

Servings: 4
Preparation time: 15 minutes

Yucca Fries
(Mandioquinha Frita)

Brazilians have many interchangeable names for what English speakers call the yucca or cassava root. Manioc, aipim, mandioca, *and* macaxeira *are just four different ways of referring to the starchy tuber that indigenous Brazilians used as the base of their food and drink. This recipe treats the essentially bland root like a potato in a rendition of oven fries. To make the fries crisp, be sure to boil the yucca first.*

> **4 cups fresh yucca, peeled, or 1 pound peeled**
> **frozen yucca**
> **Olive oil cooking spray**
> **Salt**

In a saucepan, combine the yucca with enough cold water to cover it by 1 inch. Bring the water to a boil and cook the yucca for 20 to 30 minutes, or until tender.

Preheat the oven to 375°F. With a slotted spoon transfer the yucca to a cutting board, let it cool, and cut lengthwise into 3-inch batons, discarding the thin, woody core. Spray a cookie sheet with the cooking oil. Spread the yucca batons on the cookie sheet, and spray the batons with the cooking oil. Sprinkle a little salt on top of the yucca. Bake for 8 minutes. Turn over the yucca fries and bake the other side for an additional 8 minutes.

Servings: 4–6
Preparation time: 30 minutes or less

Black Bean and Coconut Puree
(Feijão de Coco)

When you're stuck for a side dish, this easy puree can usually be scrounged up from your pantry staples. Best of all, you can prepare it in less than 10 minutes. Serve it with rice and a salad for a nutritious and tasty meal.

2 cups cooked black beans (see Note)
3 tablespoons extra-virgin olive oil
2 cloves garlic, mashed
1 onion, chopped
1 tomato, seeded and chopped
½ teaspoon salt
¼ cup Green Aroma (page 77)
½ cup coconut milk

Puree the beans in a food processor with a little bit of the soaking liquid or water.

In a skillet, sauté the garlic and onion in the olive oil over high heat. When these soften, add the tomato, salt, and Green Aroma. After one minute, add the bean puree and coconut milk, stirring the mixture rapidly as it thickens. Adjust the seasoning, adding black pepper if desired.

Servings: 10
Preparation time: 10 minutes or less

Note: You can soak dried black beans overnight and cook them for one hour, or use good-quality canned beans that have been rinsed and drained.

Seaweed Rice
(Arroz com Nori)

Make rice tastier and more nutritious by taking yet another cue from Japanese Brazilians: add seaweed and pickles. Roasted nori shreds and Japanese pickles can now be found in many supermarkets, and not just in Japanese specialty stores. If you can't find them and don't live near a Japanese grocery store, you can order these staples online (see Resources).

1 cup uncooked long-grain brown rice
4 sheets roasted teriyaki nori, torn into small strips
3 tablespoons Japanese pickled cucumber, chopped finely

Boil the rice according to its package directions. When the rice is cooked, add the nori and pickles and stir thoroughly.

Servings: 4
Preparation time: 20 minutes or less

Rice with Broccoli and Coconut
(Arroz com Broccolis)

Brazilians don't like to leave poor old rice alone. At the very least, most Brazilians sauté rice in oil and garlic before adding the cooking water, so that the rice boils up fluffy, each grain separate. To flavor rice, home cooks sometimes use a bit of coconut milk. This recipe is popular in both home cooking and at restaurants. The coconut milk adds sweetness and the broccoli adds color, flavor, and more nutrients.

> 2 cups water
> 4 tablespoons coconut milk
> 1 tablespoon olive oil
> 1 clove garlic, chopped
> 1 cup uncooked long-grain brown rice
> 1 cup fresh or frozen broccoli, chopped finely

Bring the water and the coconut milk to a boil in a lidded stockpot over high heat. As you wait for the water to boil, heat the oil in a skillet over high heat, and add the garlic. After a few seconds, add the rice and stir rapidly, making sure to coat each grain. When the garlic starts to turn golden, remove the rice from the heat. As soon as the water boils, add the rice and garlic. Reduce the heat, cover the pot, and cook for about 20 minutes, or 5 minutes less than the rice package instructs. Stir the broccoli into the rice, replace the pot lid, and cook for another 5 minutes, until all the water is completely absorbed. Fluff the rice with a fork before serving.

Servings: 6
Preparation time: 30 minutes or less

Potatoes with Nori

If you prefer potatoes to rice, try this pairing of nori and carbs.

1½ pounds new potatoes (Yukon Gold or fingerling potatoes are best),
    scrubbed and cut into quarters
2 tablespoons extra-virgin olive oil
1 cup shredded roasted nori (try *ajitsuke,* or "seasoned" nori seaweed,
    for a hot and spicy flavor)
1 tablespoon sesame seeds

Boil the potatoes in a saucepan with enough water to cover them. When tender and thoroughly cooked, drain the potatoes and dry on absorbent paper. In a large bowl, toss the potatoes with the oil. Arrange the potatoes on a serving platter, and sprinkle the nori and the sesame seeds over the potatoes while they are still hot. Toss the potatoes and serve.

Servings: 6
Preparation time: 15 minutes or less

Gnocchi with Arugula Sauce
(Nhoque com Molho de Rucola)

Brazil's substantial population of Italian ancestry has elevated gnocchi, or nhoque, to a very popular dish at lunch or dinner. While I would never dissuade anyone from making their own pasta, finding good, handmade, and fresh gnocchi has gotten easier, especially in big cities. So save the time and prepare the sauce while storebought gnocchi cooks, if you don't already have sauce at hand in the fridge.

1 (16-ounce) package freshly made gnocchi
1 cup Arugula Sauce (page 80)
¼ cup grated Parmesan or Pecorino cheese (optional)

Drop the gnocchi in boiling, salted water and cook until the pasta floats to the top and is al dente. Meanwhile, gently heat the Arugula Sauce in a saucepan over medium heat. Drain the gnocchi and place into a serving bowl. Pour the sauce over the gnocchi and toss. Serve with grated cheese over the top if you wish.

Servings: 2–4
Preparation time: 15 minutes

Cabbage Salad
(Salada de Repolho)

I remember big bowlfuls of crunchy, filling red cabbage salad always marinating in the fridge at my parents' house. For those of us looking to atone for dietary excesses, a few days of meals centered around this salad will keep you satisfied. Red cabbage has a lovely sweet taste that improves over a few days, but the dressing works equally well with savoy or white cabbage, too.

3 tablespoons sesame oil
4 tablespoons tamari
3 tablespoons rice wine vinegar
3 tablespoons mirin (Japanese rice wine)
½ teaspoon Tabasco or hot pepper sauce
1 small head red cabbage, cored and shredded

Whisk all the liquids together into an emulsion. Place the shredded cabbage in a deep bowl and toss with the dressing.

Servings: 6
Preparation time: 10 minutes or less

Hijiki Salad
(Salada de Hijiki)

At a certain Rio-based chain of barbecue houses, the salad bar is loaded with classic Japanese options, including sushi and sashimi, steamed nira (a type of chive eaten in both Brazil and Japan), and this classic seaweed salad. I often eat so much of this salad that I've little remaining appetite for devouring barbecued meat. Hijiki is sold dried, and you can now find frozen shelled edamame (soy beans) and shiitake at supermarkets. This refreshing, chewy, and healthy salad provides both nutrients and fiber.

1 (2-ounce) package dried hijiki
2 tablespoons sesame oil
1 cup sliced shiitake mushrooms
1 carrot, julienned
½ cup fresh or frozen edamame
¼ cup tamari or reduced-sodium soy sauce
3 tablespoons mirin (Japanese rice wine)

Soak the hijiki for 10 minutes in enough water to cover the seaweed.

In a skillet, heat the oil and sauté the mushrooms and carrot. Add the edamame last, and cook for another minute. Drain the hijiki and add to the skillet. Whisk the tamari and mirin together and add to the vegetables. Stir-fry for about 3 minutes, then remove from heat. Can be served hot or cold.

Servings: 4
Preparation time: 15 minutes

DESSERTS

Malted Milk Panna Cotta
(Pudim de Ovomaltine)

Fast-food behemoths like McDonald's and KFC have had notorious difficulty in rising to the top of Brazil's fast-food chain, given the idiosyncratic tastes of the population. Bob's is Brazil's version of a burger parlor. In general, I don't crave any menu items at Bob's except for one: the malted milkshake. It's reason enough to frequent Bob's and many Brazilians do that just for this frosty drink. Malted milk or Ovomaltine has always been popular in Brazil as a flavor; I struggled to find the right recipe to capture that delicate, chocolatey taste until I came up with this panna cotta pudding recipe. These puddings preserve malted milk's tangy sweetness with just the right creamy mouth-feel. I prefer to use buttermilk as it has less fat, but for real decadence, you can just use heavy cream.

⅓ cup heavy cream
1 (¼-ounce) envelope unflavored gelatin
1 vanilla pod, split
¼ cup sugar or Splenda
½ teaspoon salt
2 cups buttermilk
6 tablespoons Ovaltine or malted milk powder
6 (¾-cup) ramekins or small molds, oiled with olive oil

Place the cream in a saucepan, add the gelatin, and stir, allowing it to stand for about one minute. Then place the saucepan over medium heat and add the vanilla pod, sugar, salt, and half the buttermilk, stirring constantly while bringing the mixture to a boil. When the mixture begins to boil, turn off the heat and add the Ovaltine and the rest of the buttermilk. Scrape the inside of the softened vanilla pod into the mixture and discard the pod (or reuse it by inserting it into a sugar bowl to make vanilla sugar). Stir the mixture until integrated and thickening, and pour into the molds. Place the molds in the refrigerator and chill for at least 3 hours before serving.

To serve, pour hot water into a bowl and gently immerse the base of the molds in the hot water. Place a plate over the top of the mold and invert, allowing the panna cotta to slide out. Serve garnished with sliced strawberries or dried cherries.

Servings: 6
Preparation time: 20 minutes (not including chilling time to set)

Brazilian Fudge Balls
(Brigadeiros)

No birthday party in Brazil would be deemed complete without these fudge candies lined up daintily in frilly paper cups for the guests. You don't need a birthday party for an excuse to make them, but be sure to have enough people around to eat them. You might be tempted to devour all these little nuggets of sweet condensed milk yourself. One is more than sufficient as a sweet treat for one person.

1 (14-ounce) can sweetened condensed milk
1 tablespoon margarine
3 tablespoons high-quality Dutch-processed cocoa powder
1 cup chocolate sprinkles

In a heavy-bottomed saucepan, stir the condensed milk, margarine, and cocoa powder over medium heat. Cook the mixture until it thickens enough to show the pan's bottom when stirred. Pour the mixture in a greased glass or porcelain bowl, and let it cool to room temperature. Using two spoons, scoop small amounts of the mixture and roll between your hands to shape 1½-inch balls (rub your hands with a little margarine so the balls won't stick). Roll the balls in chocolate sprinkles to decorate. Serve the balls in decorative paper candy cups.

Servings: 20
Preparation time: 30 minutes

Açaí-Strawberry Pudding
(Pudim de Açaí e Morango)

Açaí-Strawberry Pudding makes a refreshing fruit dessert for a light meal. The tapioca's chewy note provides a fabulous texture for the sweetness of the fruit.

> 1 cup sweetened *açaí*
> 1 cup strawberries
> ½ cup sugar or Splenda
> ½ cup water
> 1 cup coconut milk
> ¼ cup organic granulated tapioca
> 1 vanilla pod, split
> 1 (¼-ounce) packet unflavored gelatin
> 1 large ring mold or 6 (¾-cup) ramekins or decorative molds, oiled
>   with olive oil

In a blender, pulse the *açaí*, strawberries, sweetener, and water together until you get a smooth mixture. Place this and the coconut milk, tapioca, and split vanilla pod in a saucepan and heat, stirring continuously. Simmer over a low flame so that the edges of the mixture bubble for about 10 minutes. Remove the vanilla pod, scraping the insides into the liquid, and add the gelatin. Stir to dissolve, then pour the mixture into the mold(s). Chill in the refrigerator to set for at least 1 hour. To remove pudding from mold(s), dip the bottom of each mold into hot water, place a serving plate on top of the mold, and invert, gently sliding the pudding onto the plate.

Servings: 6
Preparation time: 15 minutes (not including chilling time to set)

Coconut-Tapioca Pudding
(Cuscuz)

In Bahia, the best food is often served not in restaurants but in the streets. Mobile kitchens dot the squares and beaches of the region, presided over by chatty Bahiana women dressed all in white. These women, the descendents of the slaves who used resourcefulness and cunning to create Bahia's fantastic cuisine, serve delicious acarajé, moquecas, and one of my favorite sweets: cuscuz. Not to be confused with couscous, the semolina pasta of North Africa, dessert cuscuz is recognizable as a big white block of tapioca pudding covered with shreds of coconut. This snowy confection, one of many Brazilian tapioca-based sweets, is sticky and chewy but not overly sweet. That is, of course, if you can prevent the Bahiana mamas from pouring doce de leite (a liquid condensed milk sweet) on top of your slice.

2 cups coconut milk

1 cup skim milk or water

5 tablespoons sugar or Splenda

1 (6-ounce) package tapioca

1 teaspoon salt

6 tablespoons shredded coconut plus 4 tablespoons for
    garnish

Place the liquids, sweetener, and tapioca in a saucepan and cook over medium heat for about 5 minutes, or until slightly bubbling at the sides of the pan. Add the salt and stir until fully dissolved. Add 6 tablespoons of the shredded coconut, stirring as the mixture thickens—about 1 minute. Pour the liquid into a ring pan or glass casserole dish and place into the refrigerator. The pudding should be fully set after a minimum of 3 hours. Decorate the top of the pudding with the rest of the shredded coconut.

Servings: 10
Preparation time: 15 minutes (not including chilling time to set)

Pumpkin Tartlets
(Tortinhas de Abobora)

Pumpkin features as a sweet ingredient in many Brazilian recipes. Often it's served as a sticky compote. To make it more portable and decorative, I've devised a type of tart shell from phyllo pastry. You can use this phyllo base for any number of fillings both savory and sweet.

> 5 sheets phyllo dough, cut into 4 by 4-inch squares
> 3 tablespoons extra-virgin olive oil
> 1 cup diced fresh pumpkin or canned pumpkin puree
> ½ cup Splenda
> 5 whole cloves
> 1 tablespoon cinnamon
> 2 tablepoons shredded, unsweetened coconut, plus extra for garnish
> Confectioners' sugar, for sprinkling (optional)

Preheat the oven to 350°F. Brush the phyllo sheets with olive oil. Take a muffin tin and gently press two squares of phyllo dough slightly into the depressions, staggering one square at a 45-degree angle to the one beneath (making an eight-point "star"). Bake these phyllo "cups" in the oven until they turn golden and crisp slightly (about 5 to 10 minutes). Remove from the oven and the tin, and set them on a rack to cool.

If using fresh pumpkin, place the pieces into a saucepan with enough water to come halfway up the sides and cook over medium heat until soft (about 15 minutes). Mash in the pan with a fork. If using canned pumpkin, place in a saucepan.

To the pumpkin in the saucepan, add the sweetener, cloves, and cinnamon, and heat over a medium flame until thoroughly mixed and the pumpkin pulls cleanly away from the bottom when stirred. Stir in the coconut, remove the mixture from the heat, and let it cool. Remove the cloves. Spoon the mixture into the phyllo cups and serve warm with a dusting of shredded coconut or confectioners' sugar. You can also wrap the tartlets in plastic wrap and freeze, to be reheated at a later time.

Servings: 5
Preparation time: 30 minutes or less

Nut-Crusted Apple Pie
(Torta de Maçã)

Many Brazilian cakes and tarts use flour made from ground nuts, thanks to the abundance of the indigenous varieties. I remember in particular a very tasty but complicated cake my mother loved, which required ground hazelnuts. I was reminded of these nut-based desserts when I recently ate a delicious flourless apple pie from a São Paulo street vendor. Try this version, which uses dried fruit and nuts pressed together for the crust.

> 1 cup cashews
> 1½ cups walnuts
> 1 cup pitted dates
> ½ cup dried figs
> 3 apples
> Juice of 1 lemon, stirred into a bowl of water
> ½ teaspoon ground cinnamon
> ¼ teaspoon ground allspice
> ¼ teaspoon ground cloves
> 2 tablespoons Splenda or honey
> ½ cup apple juice
> ¾ cup raisins (optional)
> Yogurt (optional)
> Honey (optional)

Place the nuts, dates, and figs in a food processor and chop until the ingredients are ground and integrated, but not uniform (approximately 30 seconds). Test the mixture for texture by pinching a bit; it should be smooth and ground enough to stick together. Press this into a 9-inch tart pan. Place in a refrigerator to set while making the filling.

Core and slice the apples crosswise into ¼-inch-thick slices, then place the slices immediately in the lemon water. Drain the slices from the lemon water, then add them to a large skillet with the rest of the ingredients. If you wish to add the raisins, you can add them now. Sauté for about 10 minutes over medium heat, stirring constantly. Remove the fruit from the pan with a slotted spoon, place in a bowl, and allow it to cool.

Cook the liquid in the pan down to a syrup of approximately half the volume, then remove from the heat and allow it to cool separately.

Spread the apple slices in an even layer over the crust. Brush the syrup over the apples. Serve it right away, or store in the refrigerator for later use. Seal the tart in an airtight tub. If you desire, serve each slice with a dollop of yogurt and a small drizzle of honey.

Servings: 10–12
Preparation time: 30 minutes or less

Wobbly Marias
(Maria Mole de Limão)

Children love this refreshing green sweet, but don't let that stop you and other adults from trying it. This recipe is a nice way to introduce children to the kitchen and to enlist their help in preparing food.

½ cup water
½ cup coconut milk
1 (3-ounce) package sugar-free lime gelatin
6 tablespoons ice water
2 tablespoons extra-virgin olive oil
2 egg whites, beaten to stiff peaks
¾ cup shredded, unsweetened coconut

In a saucepan, bring the water and the coconut milk to a boil. Dissolve the gelatin in the liquid and stir rapidly. Turn off the heat. Stir in the ice water. Oil an ice-cube tray with the olive oil. Then fold the beaten egg whites into the thickening liquid and pour into the ice-cube tray. Chill in the refrigerator to set for 45 minutes, then pop the cubes out of the tray and roll them in the coconut. Serve the cubes stacked in a pyramid.

Servings: 12
Preparation time: 30 minutes or less (not including chilling time to set)

Orange Cake
(Bolo de Laranja)

My grandparents' house in Rio always held ritual treasures for me: the cool marble floors and staircases to lie on when sunburnt; the rich scent of wood and leather that lingered in my suitcase even weeks after visiting them; and the plump, sticky orange cake my grandmother always had on hand to serve my sister and me for breakfast or a snack. While I adored many things that came out of my grandmother's kitchen, that orange cake was a talisman I have spent years trying to replicate. As Brazil is the world's largest supplier of orange juice, it's no surprise that orange cakes are popular there. This one uses olive oil instead of butter, which gives it a more vegetal and delicate aroma.

2 medium-size oranges, washed and dried

Juice of ½ large orange or ½ cup orange juice

½ cup extra-virgin olive oil

1½ cups all-purpose flour

1 teaspoon baking powder

½ teaspoon baking soda

½ teaspoon salt

4 whole eggs

1½ cups sugar, Splenda, or stevia

1 teaspoon pure vanilla extract or 1 whole vanilla pod split,
    seeds and pulp scraped

½ teaspoon almond extract

3 tablespoons water

2 tablespoons Cognac (optional)

Confectioners' sugar, for dusting

Preheat oven to 350°F. Butter or oil a 9-inch round, ring, or Bundt pan. Slice off the top and bottom of the oranges and discard. Chop the oranges (including the peel) into chunks, discard seeds, and place in a food processor, pulsing the oranges while adding all the olive oil, little by little, to the orange mixture. Keep pulsing until smooth.

Sift the flour, baking powder, baking soda, and salt together.

Beat the eggs in a large bowl until they are thick, then add the sugar, vanilla, and almond extract to the eggs. Gradually add the dry ingredients to the eggs and incorporate loosely. By thirds, add the orange mixture and stir. Do not overmix. Pour into the pan and place in the oven; bake for approximately 45 minutes, or until a toothpick inserted in the center comes out clean.

While the cake bakes, put the orange juice, water and, if you wish, the Cognac into a saucepan and heat over low heat until just slightly bubbling. Allow the cake to cool on a rack before removing from the pan and placing on a round serving dish. Take a toothpick and poke several small holes into the top of the cake. Carefully pour the hot orange syrup over the top of the cake. Serve dusted with a bit of confectioners' sugar.

Servings: 12
Preparation time: 30 minutes or less (not including chilling time to set)

Coconut Flan
(Manjar de Coco)

This comforting little flan can be prepared in the morning while you drink your Automatic Pilot. Let it sit in the fridge while you're at work and you'll have a creamy dessert at the ready for the rest of the week. Prepare the Prune Compote (page 163) to go with it.

> 8 tablespoons sugar or Splenda
> Small pinch of salt
> 7 tablespoons cornstarch
> ¾ cup coconut milk
> 1 quart cold milk or buttermilk
> 5 tablespoons grated coconut

In a large saucepan, combine the sweetener, salt, and cornstarch; then pour in the coconut milk. Stir well until completely dissolved. Stir in the cold milk.

Place the pan over medium heat and boil gently for about 15 minutes, or until you get a thick cream. Stir constantly with a wood spoon as the mixture boils. Rinse a ring mold or Bundt pan in cold water and pour the cream into the pan. Let it cool, cover with plastic wrap, and refrigerate. After 4 hours or more, place a serving plate over the mold, invert, and shake gently to release the flan. Serve with Prune Compote.

Servings: 10
Preparation time: 25 minutes or less (not including chilling time to set)

Fruit Salad
(Prato do Verão)

The key to good fruit salad is color and texture. Make sure yours has reds, blues, yellows, and greens for maximum nutrition. Use whatever you can find in season but, in a pinch, frozen works well. Translated from Portuguese, prato do verão means "summer plate," due to the abundance of available colorful fruits that can be thrown into a bowl during the warmest months of the year. For a chewy note, throw in some cashews.

½ cup chopped strawberries
½ cup chopped apples
½ cup chopped mangoes (if using frozen, thaw first)
½ cup chopped melon
½ cup blueberries or raspberries
¼ cup chopped cashews
Mint or basil, for garnish

Mix all the ingredients together in a large glass bowl. If you wish, you may drizzle a little honey into salad if the fruits are not at the peak of their ripeness. Serve garnished with a sprig of mint or basil.

Servings: 6
Preparation time: 10 minutes or less

Prune Compote
(Compote de Ameixas)

Just saying the word "prune" strikes fear in the hearts of certain people. Either they hate the laxative qualities they associate with the fruit, or they simply detest its sticky, chunky texture. I tend to believe that a touch of good-quality alcohol can improve the flavor and profile of many things (not just food!), and prunes are no exception. This sophisticated fruity compote should banish any notion of the prune as candy for geriatrics. It's delicious on its own, or with a nutty topping (page 105), or served as the sauce for Coconut Flan (page 161).

2 cups fresh-squeezed orange juice
15 pitted prunes
3 tablespoons Armagnac or Cognac (optional)

In a saucepan over medium heat, bring to a boil the orange juice, prunes, and if you wish, the liquor. Then reduce the heat to low and simmer for about 15 minutes, or until the fruit is tender. Remove from heat, pour into a glass bowl, and keep covered and refrigerated.

Servings: 5
Preparation time: 20 minutes or less

Jeitinhos for Eating

"I lead a very busy life during the week and don't have the time to cook."

Jeitinho: It's true that the BBBP requires you to spend time in the kitchen. Indeed, this is time well spent, since the only way you will learn to modify your eating habits is by spending more time being directly involved preparing the food you eat. But a busy schedule can be a hindrance. The secret to managing your time more effectively lies in doing as much advance prep-work as possible for an hour or two on the weekend, and then freezing the prepared foods you've made so that you only need to defrost them as necessary. I've broken down the time and menus of the BBBP into a monthly calendar schedule of pre-prep. At first glance, the weekend pre-prep chores seem like a lot, but most of the work takes only three to fifteen minutes per item. After time, you'll be so familiar with them you'll prepare them even faster. Keep your tools clean and within easy grasp—that cuts down on your time in the kitchen. While it's always infinitely better to cook from scratch with fresh ingredients, be flexible in finding good shortcuts: Use canned beans instead of soaking; if you have to, use chopped garlic instead fresh; buy precut salad in a bag; also, some of these food items can be ordered premade and frozen (check out Resources at the back of the book).

"I want to prepare the BBBP's meals for my family, but my finicky children don't want to eat as I do."

Jeitinho: Children's palates don't necessarily jive with those of their parents. However, rather than ceding power to your children's wishes, consider compromises. A discriminating palate is cultivated over time. Children in Brazil are taught to eat everything, to appreciate diversity as well as to avoid waste. Sometimes, circumstances, such as allergies, intervene, or maybe your children are truly difficult eaters. To get your kids interested in the meals, try getting plastic food storage boxes in different shapes and sizes. Many of the program's meals involve salads and other dishes that involve multi-ingredient composition. Prepare these ingredients and set them out in the storage containers. Make meals a game whereby you allow the children to choose which components they would like to add to their own meals, rather than you dictating what they shall eat. In this way, children will feel as if they have gotten a little bit of their way, and are engaged in the process—simultaneously, this allows you to customize your meals for your family in an effort to avoid mealtime whining rather than dining.

"I hate vegetables! The BBBP is loaded with vegetables, so how can I eat this food?"

Jeitinho: People who say they hate vegetables usually have not eaten many of them prepared in different and tasty ways. Try one week of the BBBP and see how far you get eating the vegetables. Be open-minded! If you find that you are still having trouble, try to turn the vegetables you don't like into something else. For example, most people who say they hate vegetables love potatoes and pasta. So, if you don't want to eat broccoli or spinach, why not chop them up finely, add some grated potato and a beaten egg to bind them into little cakes and pan-fry them as fritters? Don't like squash, zucchini, or carrots? Use a julienne peeler to turn them into spaghetti-like strips, add a sauce of your choice, and eat it like pasta. Don't like the textures of mushrooms or kale? Cook them according to instructions, then puree them with a hand blender, add a little buttermilk and eat them as a soup. Think watercress is too peppery? Blend watercress with other vegetable leaves to make the taste milder. There are infinite ways to "disguise" vegetables and make them more appealing. Think about the things you like to eat and find ways of preparing vegetables to mimic those preparations more closely.

"I'm not a meat-eater. How can I follow the BBBP?"

Jeitinho: Brazilians are serious about meat. So a Brazilian-style diet for people who avoid animal protein can be tricky. That said, the BBBP has been structured so that the use of animal and fish protein is prepared simply (usually by grilling or roasting), and a small amount of sauce is used to flavor the protein. Reasonable-quality textured-meat substitutes can now be found in most big supermarkets and health food stores. Try grilling tempeh or textured soy protein, then use the specified sauce so as to mimic the original recipe. In the case of stews like Moqueca or Ximxim de Galinha, substitute a whole can of palm hearts and 1 cup of soy chicken for the meat portion, and follow the rest of the recipe. For salt cod dishes, substitution is a bit more difficult. If you can't eat salt cod, try to double up on another recipe instead of using the cod.

"Eating healthy food can cost a lot of money. I don't have that kind of budget. How can I follow the BBBP?"

Jeitinho: Without doubt, fast and processed food is cheaper than fresh vegetables and meat. But eating those foods only temporarily satisfies hunger; it doesn't provide you with viable nutrition. So eating cheap is a stop-gap measure. Long-term, eating like that will lead to more expensive trips to the doctor and more discomfort. You may pay less now, but you'll certainly pay more later. Buying fresh fruits and vegetables can be economical if you're careful about avoiding waste. I've tried to limit waste as much as possible in the BBBP by working in leftovers to your weekly menus, but it's only after a week or two following the shopping lists that you'll see where you need to cut waste and lower your food bills. You may also want to scrutinize your previous grocery-shopping habits. How much of your food bill went to expensive, bad-nutrition staples like sugared cereals, snacks, crackers, and more? These never come cheap, and the BBBP avoids them altogether. On the positive side, the BBBP uses a lot of beans, which are cheap and perfect for the budget conscious. Work more bean recipes into your weekly menus to keep your overall budget lower and spend on the fruits that provide a whole meal, like *açaí*.

"I've started the program but I'm finding myself hungry all the time. I want more food."

Jeitinho: In the beginning of the BBBP, adjustment to the program might involve a few days of getting used to eating less food than you might be accustomed. If you've been eating too much to begin with, lesser intake will prompt the body to ring the alarm bells by sending hunger signals to the brain. If you were starving yourself, the hunger pangs would not abate. In this case, since you are providing adequate nutrition in reasonable portions, the sensation of hunger should eventually subside. In the meantime, to make yourself more comfortable while your body adjusts, do two things: First, hydrate by drinking fluids at the right pH. Invest in a filtration water bottle (Nikken makes the best ones. See Resources.) that will make your drinking water more alkaline. Drink constantly from it throughout the day so that your body feels full. If you prefer tea to water, drinking maté also increases the sensation of fullness. Second, one trick espoused by University of California–Berkeley professor Seth Roberts—author of *The Shangri-La Diet*—seems to really work, and that is to consume one tablespoon of extra-light olive oil within a two-hour time window during which you will not ingest anything else. My clients have done this during the first week of the BBBP when they develop hunger pangs, and it works beautifully.

"I like to go out to different restaurants and don't want to just follow one style of cuisine. How can I still maintain the principles of the BBBP?"

Jeitinho: It would be unreasonable to assume that you're going to stay in every night and only eat meals that you've cooked. Eating any one cuisine all the time eventually grows tedious. When you go out to a restaurant, try to scan the menu to find a good salad to start with—preferably one with some legumes and without too much cheese or animal protein. For your main course, order a lean protein and try to combine that with at least one cruciferous vegetable (broccoli, cauliflower, kale, cabbage, and so on). Mix it up and try new foods you've never had before. As long as you follow the principle of a good lean protein, salad, and cruciferous vegetables, you're staying on the good side of the nutrition fence, even if you're going out for dinner. Of course, the BBBP also advocates having a good splurge now and then. But that means occasionally; if you're having pizza and ice cream sundaes twice a week every week, you're going to backslide to where you were before starting the BBBP.

"Making these meals involves grocery shopping and I hate grocery shopping! How can I limit my time doing that?"

Jeitinho: Luckily, you don't have to rummage through neighborhoods and phone books to find some of the more uncommon ingredients—or even the common ones—of the BBBP. Everything you need can be shopped for online (see Resources), saving you a lot of time. In some cities, you might even be able to find grocery delivery services that keep track of your purchases from week to week so that you simply check off what is dwindling in supply. To make things easier, I have emphasized the purchases of frozen products—fruits, vegetables, and more. By having a mix of canned and frozen items, you can keep your pantry stocked well enough so that your total grocery shopping time per week can be reduced to simply picking up fresh meat or vegetables.

"I have very specific dietary requirements. How can I manage my needs within the BBBP?"

Jeitinho: The BBBP is flexible enough to accommodate various dietary needs. Before you begin the BBBP, look at the menu sets for each week, then go through the recipes. Jot down the items that you are not allowed to eat. When you've finished going through the whole month's menus, go back and look at your list. If certain items keep creeping up, such as nuts or eggs or sugar (the usual culprits), see where you can take them out altogether or substitute (many health food stores carry egg substitutes, and stevia is a good sugar substitute). Go back to your list and identify the recipes that you can eat.

Then redraw a menu schedule, using the BBBP as a rough outline, listing only the recipes you can make. Fill in the gaps by seeking recipes that work on a similar principle as the BBBP: to make a meal, eat a lean protein with a little bit of a concentrated sauce; a salad of legumes; and plenty of fruit and vegetables.

"I can't cook. How can I follow the program?"

Jeitinho: Think of this as an opportunity to learn. If you can operate a blender, boil water, chop vegetables, and turn on a stove, you can make more than half of the recipes. Very few dishes involve complicated cooking technique, so as long as you follow the instructions, you shouldn't have too much difficulty. Start small and work your way up to trickier recipes as you build up your confidence. Bean salads, sauces, salads, and grilled meats (this is where having a portable griller in the kitchen might come in handy) should be in your first tier of preparation—some don't even require cooking. Get through those then try making some of the stews, like Ximxim de Galinha and Moqueca. Save for last making more complicated dishes like fritters and desserts. Get a little notebook. Each time you make a new dish, note what could be improved. With practice, you'll find that fear of cooking needn't be an impediment to learning and, ultimately, doing it.

5

Se Mexe!
("Move It!"):
The Exercises

On Movement

BRAZILIANS love to move.

Soccer, or *futebol,* is the most visible and famous manifestation of Brazilian athleticism, but it is by no means the only one. Such sports as volleyball, jiu-jitsu, and judo consume the nation's attention, and the country has repeatedly spawned world champions and Olympic gold medal–winners in each of these three pursuits. Surfing and body-boarding—beach activities tailor made for the Brazilian population—also have their share of Brazilian national and world champions. These six sports are beloved and pursued by the average Brazilian.

Brazilians are lucky. Because of their climate and geography, they have plenty of incentives to keep motivated and active. When you live in a tropical country with big beaches, forests, and mountains, staying fit to enjoy yourself as well as to look good becomes second nature. Brazilians like to look good. Fancy gyms and Pilates studios dot street corners in the larger cities to the same degree that they do in style-obsessed cities like New York and Los Angeles.

Observers might describe Brazilians (especially the urbanites) as uniquely vain, pointing to their obsessions with bodies—especially the buttocks—and their world-famous plastic surgeons. I would argue that Brazilians are body-conscious simply because their bodies are on display more often than in other cultures.

The Bottom Line: Brazilians and Body Image

In comparison to Brazilians, those who live in regions where climate requires remaining covered up tend to experience body-consciousness as self-consciousness. To take an important example: If you're like the great majority of the population, you probably hate your bottom, and spend a fair amount of time worrying self-consciously about it. Chances are, your exercise motivation has been a pursuit to shape your butt, or minimize it as much as possible.

In Brazil, a land where the tropical climate dictates a minimum of clothing, the *bunda,* or *bum bum* (the affectionate and ubiquitous Portuguese terms for the rear end), is king. In fact, it is positively glorified in all aspects of the culture, whether it's being

A TINY AND INCOMPLETE LIST OF BRAZILIAN ATHLETES

Soccer
- Manuel Francisco dos Santos (Garrincha): Member of winning World Cup squads of 1958 and 1962
- Edson Arantes de Nascimento (Pelé): Record-breaking member of winning World Cup squads of 1958, 1962, and 1970
- Jair Ventura Filho (Jairzinho): Member of 1970 winning World Cup squad
- Arthur Antunes Coimbra (Zico): 1983 Player of the Year
- Ronaldinho: FIFA World Player of the Year 2004 and 2005

Formula One Racing
- Emerson Fittipaldi: World Champion 1972 and 1974
- Nelson Piquet: World Champion 1981, 1983, and 1987
- Ayrton Senna: World Champion 1988, 1990, and 1991

Volleyball
- Men's national team: World Champions 2003; Champion of the League 2003; Olympic gold medalists 1992; silver medalists 1984
- Women's national team: Olympic bronze medalists 1992; five-time title-holders of the Grand Prix 1994, 1996, 1998, 2004, and 2005

Brazilian Jiu-Jitsu
- Three generations of the Gracie family: Legendary fighting family and progenitors of Brazilian jiu-jitsu

Tennis
- Gustavo Kuerten (Guga): Winner of the French Open 1997, 2000, and 2001

Skateboarding
- Bob Burnquist: Winner of X-Games 2001

shown off on a beach, displayed on television and billboard advertising, or featured in song, film, or literature.

It would be safe to say that Brazilians are obsessed with the *bunda*, and use the term daily, without self-consciousness. That same lack of self-consciousness pervades the individual attitudes that people have about their own bodies; a fact that can be plainly witnessed on any beach. Buttocks of every size and shape walk unashamedly in bikinis that resemble little more than a couple of strings, attached to owners who may be thin or fat, smooth or dimpled, young or old. Brazil may be famous for the vanity of its citizens, but paradoxically, that self-regard is benevolent in that it encompasses as wide a continuum of shapes and sizes as possible.

The fact is, Brazilians love a well-rounded bottom. Polls in the country regarding sexuality suggest that the casual attitudes toward physical shapes and sizes yield a more happy and satisfied population, especially in the sexual department. In fact, an Italian research survey by the magazine *Riza Psicosomatica* identified Brazilians as actually spending significantly more time engaging in sex than do the people of any other nation. No wonder an international poll of Club Med goers ranked Brazilians as the hottest nationality. It's not just about the physical presence, it's really about the attitude you project with regard to your physical presence. If you're proud of what you've got, whether it's small, big, orange-peeled, or firm, you'll project a more confident nature that in turn translates into contentedness.

It's easy to forget this when you live in countries where the body ideal projected by the media is one of unattainable slimness. While being overweight to the degree that one cannot move oneself easily is never attractive or healthy, neither is neurotic, celebrity-style boniness, either. It is evolutionarily hard-wired into our genes to desire healthy bodies that are not starving or weak. I want to emphasize that this in no way advocates being overweight as a positive choice. The attendant illnesses of obesity—diabetes, heart disease, back pain, liver dysfunction, arthritis, etc.—are neither attractors nor keys to a better life. But being healthy and accepting your body shape within a framework of eating well and daily movement certainly are. In the end, the level of pleasure you take from the body you inhabit is mostly in the mind.

The truth is, you can tone the muscles of the buttocks to a certain degree, including the three main gluteals—gluteus medius, gluteus minimus, and gluteus maximus. With proper nutrition and targeted exercise, you can slim your buttocks to an extent, but the shape with which you are born tends to dictate how much can actually change. If that means you are pear-shaped in the way that Jennifer Lopez or Beyoncé Knowles have so effectively exploited to their advantage (a shape that defines a majority of women), no matter how much you exercise or diet, short of starving yourself, you will not have the flat backside of a supermodel.

For your own health and sanity, try discarding hang-ups you may have about what you may perceive to be "faults" or "flaws" in your appearance. Chances are, you might be more bothered by them than anyone else. But think of it this way: With every passing day, you are going to get older. That's a fact. Following that logic, you will never look as good in the future as you do today. So capitalize on it! What you eat and how you move will always have a more long-lasting impact on your looks than any creams, potions, or even cosmetic procedures, so take the time now to start a program like the BBBP to improve your body and mind as a holistic unit.

Making the Effort

Heat and landscape would be enough to naturally drive any population into bathing suits and out into the sand and surf, to show off those butts. But Brazilians have a definitive national zest for activity that orients them so much more to movement. It's one way in which Brazilians express a unified vitality and power, perhaps as a psychological reaction to the domestic problems that persist and continue to oppress so many.

It's worth taking a cue from Brazilians on energy and movement, particularly as it concerns your own health.

For optimal well-being (and to look your best), you must add consistent and daily vigorous movement to your life. The key is in maintaining a certain amount of intensity. In 2006, researchers from Canada's University of Alberta disclosed the results of a clinical study to the American College of Sports Medicine; they found that low-intensity activity, such as walking, was not providing health benefits to practitioners, especially in comparison to those who pursued slightly tougher workouts. "Gentle" exercise isn't enough to make significant changes in your fitness and weight. Similarly, eating food only in small, low-calorie portions does not suffice if you wish to lose weight long-term. Without a movement plan tethered to an eating plan, you'll inevitably mire yourself in cycles of binging and starving. You will constantly scrutinize your meals for caloric content—whether consciously or unconsciously. This is no way to enjoy life.

So let's say you've figured out how to integrate the BBBP's eating plan into your life. To arrive at a good physique that's genetically right for you, you must be active to the point at which you burn as many or slightly more calories than those you consume. While the math may be simple, doing it isn't. Even the best athletes require more than self-motivation to stay on the right track—a fact to which thousands of personal trainers and coaches can attest.

Exercise has to be interesting, and it must achieve a balance between a degree of difficulty that is just hard enough for the workout to be a challenge, but not so difficult as to prevent less active people from taking part. The BBBP's movement plan achieves this by fusing a fascinating, uniquely Brazilian form of movement with a century-old international fitness phenomenon that has found an unusually receptive following in Brazil.

The Movement Plan

The BBBP's movement plan brings together elements of capoeira, the Brazilian martial art, with exercises from Pilates, the fitness regimen developed one hundred years ago by the German boxer and acrobat Joseph Pilates. In deference to both disciplines, I must emphasize that this movement plan is a distinct hybrid. As a student and practitioner of both these complex activities, I urge people to understand the fundamental difference between both practices in their pure forms, and the use of some of their aspects within the BBBP's movement plan.

Combining elements of the two disciplines makes a lot of sense, because they are very complementary. Capoeira and Pilates both require strength and propulsion from the lower abdominal and back muscles. Movements in both must be initiated from the core of the body and extend outward to the peripheries of the limbs. Capoeira demands speed, agility, and power; Pilates optimizes the body's ability to deliver all three. Both emphasize total focus and concentration, establishing a connection between the mind and the body. Together, the basics of these two practices increase balance and stability; articulate the spine and attenuate the muscles, giving practitioners a longer, leaner look; heighten the sense of strength, control, and mastery over one's body; and, consequently, leave exercisers feeling rejuvenated and exhilarated.

LEANDRO CARVALHO

A fitness instructor for seventeen years, Leandro Carvalho is the creator of the "Brazilian" series of workouts featured at the Equinox Fitness Clubs, a national chain of luxury gyms headquartered in New York City. A physical education graduate of Minas Gerais College with a master's degree in recreation/dance therapy from New York University, Carvalho was also a dancer with the Merce Cunningham Dance Company.

An example of Brazil leading the way in fitness is in aerobics competitions. The country has had several world champions in aerobics. A lot of dancers and gymnasts in Brazil have very short careers. Brazil has a passion for music, for dance, for fitness. And I think because we are so very musical, and dancing is in our blood, aerobics is easy for us. That's why we are champions: We can do all the jumps!

In the fitness world in New York, being Brazilian has always helped me. For one thing, it has always brought me other Brazilian clients who want to stay fit, many of whom have worked with me for years. Even now, I teach Brazilians, like the Victoria's Secret models.

But things went really crazy in 2000, when all of a sudden there was this Latin explosion, with J. Lo and Ricky Martin. Latin music and dance became very "in." I was around at the right time, and came up with the right proposal. All the New York clubs wanted Brazilian classes. So I started teaching four classes a day, and they were packed! Now I teach a total of seven Brazilian-style classes: Brazilian Body Surf, Brazilian Bodysculpt, Brazilian Butt-Lift, Brazilian Groove, Brazilian Stretching, Brazilian Tummy-Tuck, and Brazilian Upper-Cuts. I was really happy when New York magazine voted my classes as the best ones in the city.

Teaching this much means I have to eat every two hours. I stay very tough on that. I eat things like oatmeal with almond milk, some bananas, and blueberries, and I try to mix in a little protein powder into fruit shakes. I also drink açaí and coconut milk. It's better to eat varied foods like that. I enjoy it and it's good for you. It's certainly more fun than dieting. I'm also trying to eat more Brazilian food than I did before. I try to eat a lot of vegetables, fruits, and fish, and keep things varied. I don't eat as much red meat as Brazilians do, but I still eat it. I am Brazilian, after all.

Capoeira

The repercussions of slavery's cruel history in Brazil echo today in the form of capoeira.

From approximately 1532 to 1888, more than 3 million people were abducted from their homes all over Africa and enslaved in Brazil to harvest sugarcane, one of the most dangerous and back-breaking of all farming jobs. They suffered squalid living conditions among people from different tribes and countries who spoke different languages; tension was constant; violence was rife.

Historians assume that until the first decade of the nineteenth century, capoeira was tolerated by the Portuguese, Dutch, and French masters as a way of reducing tensions among the slaves. The colonists reasoned that ritualized fights served as escape valves for the daily pressure in slaves' lives. The slave-owners reckoned that allowing capoeira kept Africans submissive by focusing their aggression on each other.

Because very few written records on capoeira before 1814 exist, the origins and traditional rituals of capoeira remain murky. According to conventional wisdom, capoeira was practiced mostly in Recife, Rio de Janeiro, and Bahia—where it probably originated. Capoeira most likely began as a synthesis of traditional African dances and pugilism, accompanied by musical instruments, and was probably one of the few opportunities for slaves to express themselves and their culture.

In 1808, the Portuguese King Dom João IV moved his royal seat and the court to Brazil to flee Napoleon Bonaparte's invasion of Portugal, and capoeira was no longer tolerated. Records of arrests of slaves practicing capoeira turn up as early as 1821. Nervous Portuguese governors could see that capoeira was becoming a unifying force among Africans, generating expert fighters, and wounding valuable workers—three very threatening developments. By 1892, capoeira was completely banned from Brazil.

But like all once-sanctioned pursuits, capoeira continued to be practiced in secret. By 1888, when slavery in Brazil was officially abolished, capoeira entered a period of *malandragem* (roguery). The best fighters used capoeira for violent and nefarious ends. Though capoeira is traditionally referred to as a game, and sparring is always described as "playing," the early 1900s saw regular, bloody displays of capoeira among criminal gangs.

Two Styles of Capoeira

In 1932, the tide began to turn for capoeira and its future. Manuel dos Reis Machado, also known as Mestre (Master) Bimba, opened his Centro de Cultura Fisica Regional Baiano, the first capoeira academy, in Salvador, Bahia. Bimba was a legendary figure who established the regional school of capoeira, a style associated with an aggressive warrior spirit and an attitude of "brain over brawn." Then–Brazilian president Getulio Vargas encouraged Bimba, believing that harnessing capoeira as a force for good by teaching it as a national sport would instill discipline, especially among young people.

In 1941, Vicente Ferreira Pastinha, also known as Mestre Pastinha, opened his own school, which taught another variant of the game, capoeira Angola. The capoeira Angola school taught a more intuitive, improvisational style of capoeira.

Today, the two schools represent the dual sides of capoeira. The legacies of Bimba and Pastinha, widely recognized as the most important figures in capoeira history, have propelled capoeira out of an exclusive association with vice to one of Brazil's most vital native forms of expression.

Capoeira's flowing, constant movement links defensive escape positions with rapid standing and rotational kicks, sweeping moves, and gymnastic cartwheels, flips, and headspins. Two players spar within a *roda* ("circle" or "wheel"), its perimeter formed by other players standing, clapping, singing traditional capoeira songs and accompanying play with sounds from the three traditional instruments: the *berimbau*, a long bow attached to a gourd that is struck by a wooden stick, dictating the rhythm of the *roda*'s action; the *atabaque*, a tall wooden hand drum; and the *pandeiro*, a type of tambourine. Tradition requires *capoeiristas* to have talent not only playing within the *roda*, but to demonstrate equal skill in playing the instruments and singing the traditional songs that accompany play.

Much nuance colors capoeira. Success lies in balancing openness, sympathy, and clever, strategic attack. It takes years to become proficient in capoeira, as with any martial art. But capoeira is more than a fight, dance, or game; it's a political statement born of oppression; it's a way of connecting, or developing awareness of the wider world around you; it's a physical activity designed to engage body and brain.

The BBBP workouts incorporate the most basic actions of capoeira to raise the heart rate and help practitioners develop balance, control, and agility. Capoeira serves as an excellent complement to Pilates-based movement, the other component of the BBBP exercise plan.

Pilates

Joseph Pilates was perhaps the greatest fitness visionary of the twentieth century. In his 1934 book *Your Health: A Corrective System of Exercising that Revolutionizes the Entire Field of Physical Education*, he defined his method as "the science and art of coordinated body-mind-spirit development through natural movements under strict control of the will." The method harnesses six key components: breath, concentration, centering oneself from what Pilates called "the powerhouse" (the group of muscles that encircle the lower trunk and pelvis), precision, flowing movement, and control.

Pilates was frequently ridiculed by members of the medical establishment of his day— a fact that caused him much sadness and frustration. Now, decades after his death in 1967, scientists with more advanced technology and understanding of biomechanics confirm what Pilates knew all along: For optimal health, the best results come from a holistic approach to core conditioning of the lower abdominals and pelvis—the region that supports the spine and the nerve impulses that go from the brain to all the muscles of the body.

Joseph Hubertus Pilates was born in Germany in 1880. Riddled with serious health problems, Pilates was bedridden for the better part of his first ten years. Seized by a ferocious will to overcome his infirmities, he avidly read as many books as he could on anatomy, kinesiology, classical Greco-Roman movement, and Asian disciplines such as yoga and various martial arts. The system of conditioning he derived from piecing together all this knowledge was so potent that by the age of fourteen he had recovered sufficiently from his own debilities to become a well-known boxer, acrobat, and model for medical texts. He left Germany to travel around Europe with a circus as a resident strongman and tumbler, and eventually found himself in England.

During World War I, while interned at a prison camp on the Isle of Man in the United Kingdom, he used his system of conditioning—which he called Contrology, or "The Art of Control"—to treat the sick and wounded at the camp. His method was so effective that when the great influenza pandemic of 1918 raged through Europe and killed two-thirds of the people in the camp, none of the prisoners who practiced Pilates' method died.

After the war, word of Pilates' method reached members of Germany's rising political leaders. Pilates was asked to train members of the German police in his technique. He returned to his native country, but fearing the implications, Pilates decided to go to New York City, where he opened his first studio on Manhattan's Eighth Avenue in 1926.

During the studio's first two decades, the clientele was predominantly male. As a boxer, Joe attracted other men like him who appreciated his gruff and no-nonsense workout style. In the '40s, however, the studio and the method began attracting New York's dance world elite—most famously, the choreographers George Balanchine and Martha Graham, who referred injured dancers who could benefit from Pilates' reparative and strengthening qualities. In the studio, practitioners made use of the extraordinary equipment Pilates invented and built—and apparatus-work still forms the heart of Pilates today.

Toward the end of Pilates' life, when he was no longer able to carry on teaching and maintaining the studio, the duties of carrying on Pilates' technique were transferred to a very small group of staunch loyalists, many of whom had—like the man himself—overcome injuries by training in the method.

It's only been within the last decade that Pilates has grown from being mainly a New York–centric fitness secret among cognoscenti to a global craze. Interestingly, Brazil has taken up Pilates in a much more avid manner than almost any other place in the world outside of the United States. In Ipanema alone, a district far less than half the size of Manhattan, I've counted over twenty Pilates studios. That's almost the number of studios in all of Manhattan itself!

Pilates' popularity lies in how the Brazilian medical and physiotherapeutic community support it. Indeed, Pilates instructors tend to come to the discipline as a secondary career after having become licensed physiotherapists. The primary reason behind Pilates' popularity in Brazil, apart from the fact that it keeps regulars in bikini-ready shape, is its malleability: It benefits the healthy and the injured, the young and the old, and, of course, both men and women.

The BBBP uses key Pilates mat-work sequences. Traditionally, Pilates moves the body from a horizontal position (where gravity exerts the least effect on the muscles) at the start of a session, to finish with the body in a vertical position. The BBBP workouts depart from this slightly in that they move the exercisers from horizontal to vertical position several times in the course of the workout. This is done to maximize the aerobic quality of the work.

Before You Begin

There are three BBBP workouts: the Mini Workout, the Half-Hour Workout, and the Full-Hour Workout. The thirty-day program (see page 52) lets you know which day to do which workout. However, if your personal schedule makes this difficult, try to work out a minimum of three times a week, even if all you can cram in is a Mini Workout upon waking or before bed. As you do the workouts, always remember to keep your abdominals engaged by lifting them in and up. Wear comfortable clothing that isn't too loose, use socks or work in bare feet, and use a thick exercise or Pilates mat (yoga mats are too thin).

BEFORE YOU START

Consult a doctor before undertaking this nutrition and movement program. Your medical history and current fitness status must be considered before attempting these exercises. Adjust workouts to suit your stamina, mobility, or injury levels.

Work your way up gradually. If you haven't exercised in a while, try the 10-minute Mini Workout once or twice a day every day until you can manage the Full-Hour Workout.

Don't get discouraged. If performing these moves for the first time, you will be unable to execute them all perfectly in your first few attempts. Keep working at it at a measured and steady pace so that you develop a "muscle-memory" of the movement.

Eliminate negative preconceptions about your abilities. Be positive about your movement: If you constantly reinforce the idea that you're inflexible or uncoordinated by assuming it's a fixed state, your body will have a much harder time reversing the situation. Instead, always assume the potential for improvement.

Above all, move. Aim to refine your precision in the exercises over time. Even if you flub a few movements, keep going in order to maintain an elevated heart rate.

Fuel up. The Full-Hour Workout can burn up to 700 calories when done at speed by a veteran practitioner, so make sure your body can work at its best. Make sure to eat a little something (select from the Small Bites menu in chapter 3) at least half an hour before you exercise.

Hydrate before and after workouts. Keep a bottle of water or coconut water within reach while you exercise, and be sure to drink plenty—at least a liter—when you've finished.

WHILE WORKING OUT

Engage your abdominals. Don't allow the belly to "hang out." Aim to keep your abdominals lifted in and up throughout the course of the entire workout. Initiate your movement from the core and always extend outward toward the extremities. Never let your belly flare outward or arch your spine, especially when on your back.

Breathe! Pay close attention to the breath cues as outlined in the exercise descriptions. In general, inhalation occurs when the body is being extended or stretching out; exhalation occurs during and aids flexion, when the body is folding in on itself. DON'T hold on to your breath at any time during the exercises. It should flow as continually as your movement.

Keep all four limbs retracted into the joint sockets of the torso for maximum stability (the legs root into the hip sockets and the arms root into the shoulder sockets). At the same time you draw the limbs into the sockets, try to extend the tips of the extremities (the heels of the feet and the fingertips) away in opposition from the joint sockets to stretch the muscles. Do this whether you are standing, seated, supine, or prone.

Keep your shoulders on your back. Be aware of hunching. Remember to constantly draw your shoulders away from your ears and lift the crown of your head to keep your neck long on the spine.

Anchor the body. If standing, root your feet into the floor by spreading your weight across the four corners of both feet. If on your back, the four corners of your supine body—the two hip bones and the two base tips of the shoulder blades—should be firmly planted into the floor.

Maintain control and flow. Avoid all herky-jerky movements. Avoid using momentum. "Throwing" yourself into a movement is a cheat, breaks up flow, and can cause injury.

Move with grace and power. By performing the Brazilian Bikini Body Program, you will acquire greater balance and strength over time. But as you get there, even when you are learning the exercises, avoid halfhearted movement. Stay lifted and anchored no matter where your body is, and execute the movement to the best of your ability with intent. Aim to maintain the poetry-in-motion qualities of capoeira and Pilates by keeping your transitions fluid from one exercise into the next.

FOR BEGINNERS, THE INJURED, AND SPECIAL CASES

Beginners: Use the Safety Note modifications if you lack the requisite abdominal strength to perform the movements as outlined. After three workouts with modifications, try again and leave them out, to see if you've gained enough strength to proceed at the next level.

Hamstring tightness: Keep your knees soft with a very slight bend. When doing exercises that involve being seated upright (e.g., Spine-Stretch Forward, the Saw), you may fold a small towel under your buttocks to lift your hips an inch or two off the floor to permit leg extension without gripping the hip flexors.

Knee injuries: Always maintain legs in a parallel stance and avoid locking or hyperextending your legs at the joints. Keep your knees soft.

Neck or shoulder injuries: Keep your head on the mat during supine exercises.

Pregnant: Make sure to consult with your obstetrician before undertaking this type of movement program. In general, only women who have had at least six months of Pilates experience prior to becoming pregnant should undertake the program. If you decide to perform the workouts, be careful about continuing to do the program beyond the first trimester. All prone exercises are contraindicated.

Post partum: Wait a minimum of six weeks before undertaking this movement program. Consult your doctor first to ensure that no underlying conditions will be aggravated by vigorous core work.

The Mini Workout

DURATION: Approximately 10 minutes

Exercise 1: **Ginga**
Exercise 5: **The Hundred**
Exercise 6: **Roll-Ups**
Exercise 7: **Single-Leg Circles**
Exercise 8: **Rolling Like a Ball**
Exercise 10: **Single-Leg Stretch**
Exercise 11: **Double-Leg Stretch**
Exercise 12: **Single Straight-Leg Stretch (the Scissors)**
Exercise 13: **Double Straight-Leg Stretch (the Lower-Lift)**
Exercise 14: **Criss-Cross**
Exercise 1: **Ginga**
Exercise 31: **Roll-Down with Plank Push-Ups**
Exercise 32: **Balance Finish**

The Half-Hour Workout

DURATION: Approximately 30 minutes

Exercise 1: **Ginga**
Exercise 5: **The Hundred**
Exercise 6: **Roll-Ups**
Exercise 7: **Single-Leg Circles**
Exercises 2, 3, and 4: **Ginga com 3 Esquivas (Swinging to Dodge from the Rear, from the Front, and from the Side)**
Exercise 8: **Rolling Like a Ball**
Exercise 10: **Single-Leg Stretch**
Exercise 11: **Double-Leg Stretch**
Exercise 12: **Single Straight-Leg Stretch (the Scissors)**
Exercise 13: **Double Straight-Leg Stretch (the Lower-Lift)**
Exercise 14: **Criss-Cross**
Exercise 9: **Ginga com Negativa e Rolê**
Exercise 15: **Spine-Stretch Forward**
Exercise 18: **The Saw**
Exercise 19: **Swan Prep**

Exercise 20: **Single-Leg Kick**

Exercise 21: **Double-Leg Kick**

Exercise 1: **Ginga**

Exercise 32: **Balance Finish**

The Full-Hour Workout

DURATION: Approximately 1 hour

Exercise 1: **Ginga**

Exercises 2, 3, and 4: **Ginga com 3 Esquivas (Swinging to Dodge from the Rear, from the Front, and from the Side)**

Exercise 5: **The Hundred**

Exercise 6: **Roll-Ups**

Exercise 7: **Single-Leg Circles**

Exercise 8: **Rolling Like a Ball (Rocking up to Standing)**

Exercise 9: **Ginga com Negativa e Rolê (Swinging into Low Crouch and Roll)**

Exercise 10: **Single-Leg Stretch**

Exercise 11: **Double-Leg Stretch**

Exercise 12: **Single Straight-Leg Stretch (the Scissors)**

Exercise 13: **Double Straight-Leg Stretch (the Lower-Lift)**

Exercise 14: **Criss-Cross**

Exercise 1: **Ginga**

Exercise 15: **Spine-Stretch Forward**

Exercise 16: **Modified Open-Leg Rocker**

Exercise 17: **Corkscrew**

Exercise 18: **The Saw**

Exercise 9: **Ginga com Negativa e Rolê**

Exercise 19: **Swan Prep**

Exercise 20: **Single-Leg Kick**

Exercise 21: **Double-Leg Kick**

Exercise 22: **Neck-Pull with Around the World**

Exercise 23: **Shoulder-Bridge**

Exercise 24: **Side Series—Side Kicks**

Exercise 25: **Side Series—Hip Circles**

Exercise 26: **Side Series—Leg Lifts**

Exercise 27: **Ginga com Bênção (Swinging with "Blessing" Kick)**

Exercise 28: **Teaser**

Exercise 29: **Swimming**

Exercise 30: **Seal**

Exercises 2, 3, and 4: **Ginga com Esquivas**

Exercise 31: **Roll-Down with Plank Push-Ups**

Exercise 32: **Balance Finish**

1. GINGA (Swinging)

Set-up Plant your feet hip-width apart and parallel. Keep your knees bent and the weight of your body centered through the balls of your feet.

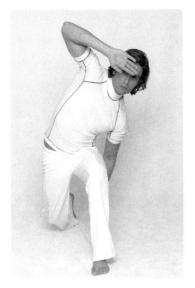 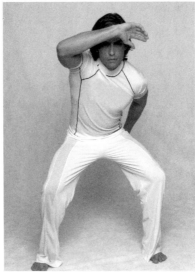 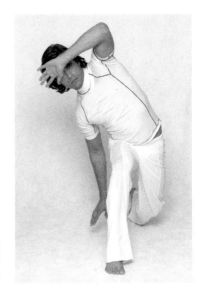

Action

1. Face forward and extend your right leg behind you, pressing back onto the ball of your right foot. Bend your knee in a slight lunge, keeping the top of that knee over your left second toe for maximum stability. Raise your right arm up to defend your face as you swing your left arm behind you for balance.

2. Bring your right leg forward to come parallel to the left leg but keep your feet slightly further than hip-width apart. Keep your center of gravity low by engaging your abdominals, leaning your upper body forward, and tucking your pelvis under as if you were about to sit down.

3. Extend your left leg back as you lunge, pressing onto the ball of your left foot, and bend your right knee over the right second toe. Now raise your left arm to defend your face as you swing your right arm back.

Move fluidly to connect the movements, swaying rhythmically from one side to the other. Keep the movement vigorous, sitting into your pelvis as you lunge. You should be drawing an "X" pattern with your legs as you ginga.

Repeat 10 full times, alternating between 10 lunges on the left and 10 lunges on the right.

2. GINGA COM ESQUIVA PRA TRÁS (Swinging to Dodge from the Rear)

Set-up Continue to ginga and prepare to dodge or "escape" defensively to the rear.

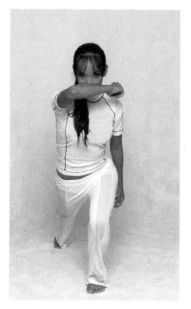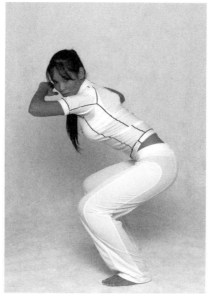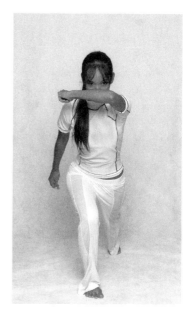

Action

1. Face forward and extend your right leg behind you, pressing back onto the ball of your right foot. Bend your left knee in a slight lunge, keeping the top of that knee over your left second toe for maximum stability. Raise your right arm up to defend your face as you swing your left arm behind you for balance.

2. Rotate your body to the right and crouch low, sitting into your pelvis and pivoting your feet to a parallel stance. Your left arm comes up to defend your face as your right arm defends the back of your head. Your head and eyes should be turned forward. In the Esquiva, your back should be almost parallel to the floor. To exit the Esquiva, rotate your knees forward to face front, with your right leg back in the lunge and your front knee bent forward. Raise your right arm to defend your face and swing your left arm back.

3. Bring your right leg forward and shift your weight to ginga and draw your left leg back. Continue to ginga as you dodge defensively on both sides.

Repeat 10 full times, alternating between 10 Esquivas pra Trás on each side. Ginga completely on both sides before each Esquiva.

3. GINGA COM ESQUIVA DA FRENTE (Swinging to Dodge from the Front)

Set-up Continue to ginga and prepare to dodge or "escape," defensively facing forward.

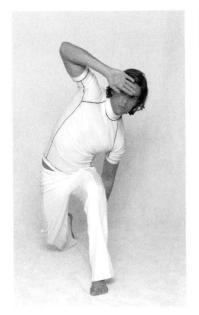 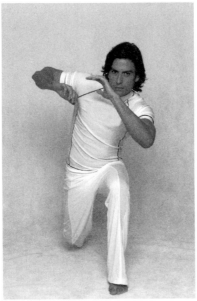 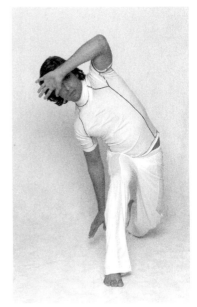

Action

1. Face forward and extend your right leg behind you, pressing onto the ball of the right foot. Bend the left knee in a slight lunge, keeping the top of your left knee over your left second toe for maximum stability. Raise your right arm up to defend your face as you swing your left arm behind you for balance.

2. Bend your right knee down to just one inch above the floor. Draw your upper body over the left thigh as you defend your face with the right arm. Lean into your left side and sit into your pelvis as you keep your abdominals drawn in and up. Don't let your belly hang over your leg!

3. Lift your body from the Esquiva and step your right foot forward to parallel with your left. Extend your left leg back and continue to ginga. Alternate legs as you attempt the Esquiva da Frente, leaning into the side of your forward leg.

Repeat 10 full times, alternating between 10 Esquivas da Frente on each side. Ginga completely on both sides before each Esquiva.

4. GINGA COM ESQUIVA LATERAL (Swinging to Dodge from the Side)

Set-up Continue to ginga and prepare to dodge or "escape" defensively to the side.

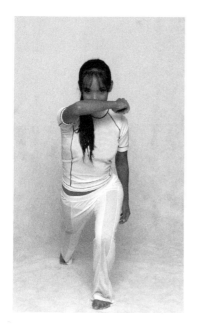 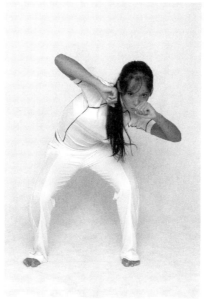 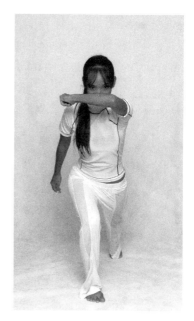

Action

1. Face forward and extend your right leg behind you, pressing onto the ball of your right foot. Bend your left knee in a slight lunge, keeping the top of your left knee over your left second toe for maximum stability. Raise your right arm up to defend your face as you swing your left arm behind you for balance.

2. Bring your right foot forward so that it is parallel to your left. Lean your upper body to your left side and over your left thigh as you defend your face with your right arm. Keep your abdominals drawn in and up. Crouch low and sit into your pelvis.

3. Lift your body from the Esquiva and cross your left foot back to continue the ginga. Alternate sides as you attempt the Esquiva Lateral.

Repeat 10 full times, alternating between 10 Esquivas Lateral on each side. Ginga completely on both sides before each Esquiva.

5. THE HUNDRED

Set-up Center yourself in an upright position, your feet parallel and hip-width apart. Cross your arms genie-style, keeping your shoulders on your back and lifting your abdominals in and up. Cross one leg over the other and lower yourself to the floor without sticking your buttocks out. Gently lie on the floor and center yourself again by taking a deep breath in through your nose and exhaling strongly as you draw your abdominals in and up.

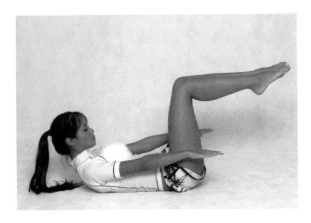

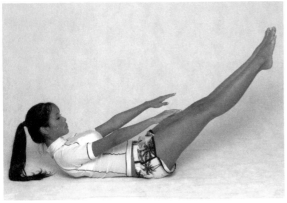

Action

1. Bring your knees into your chest, then bring your shoulders up and forward to draw your chin into your chest. Extend your arms, keeping your fingers long and your shoulders on your back. The base of your shoulder blades at both the right and left corners should be firmly anchored to the floor, as should your right and left hip bones and your tailbone.

2. Extend your legs out to a 45-degree angle, keeping your feet parallel and soft. Pump your arms vigorously up and down as you breathe in for 5 counts, then breathe out for 5 counts. As you work, make sure your arms are long and straight—no flapping at the wrist. On each exhale, expand your body through your ribs on each side, see if you can scoop your belly in and up a little deeper each time.

Do 10 breaths for a total of 100 counts.

Safety Note: *If you cannot keep your legs extended at an angle during the Hundred, you can keep your legs bent with your feet on the floor, or keep your legs in a tabletop position (knees bent at 90 degrees, directly over your hips, shins parallel to the floor), or lift them straight up toward the ceiling—in ascending order of difficulty.*

In addition, if you can't keep your shoulders lifted and chin toward your chest while on your back, keep your head on the floor. This goes for all exercises in a supine position that require the shoulders to be lifted and the chin tucked into the chest.

6. ROLL-UPS

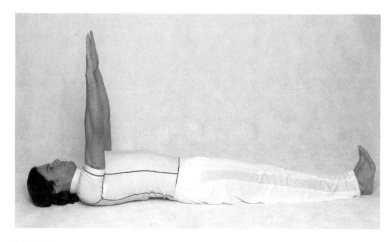

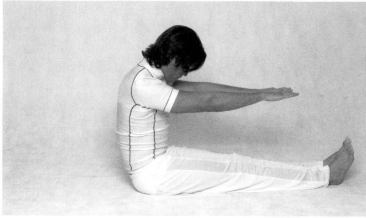

Set-up Extend your legs onto the floor. "Zipper up" the legs, drawing your shins, knees, and thighs together, and rotate the tops of your upper thighs inward. Flex your feet, using your inner thighs to extend the heels and balls of your feet away from your hips, thereby lengthening your legs. Draw your arms up toward the ceiling and retract them back fully into your shoulders. You should feel the tops of the blades pressing into the floor, anchoring yourself into your four corners.

Action

1. Inhale as you draw your head through your arms, and peel your back up off the floor one vertebra at a time. Roll your spine up and forward continuously with control and no jerking movements. Keep your arms at shoulder-height. When your body has rolled up midway, exhale and reach your fingertips past your toes. Keep your arms at shoulder-height and your shoulders on your back! Your body should be in a rounded curve, head down with a fist-length distance between your chin and your chest, arms reaching forward as your abdominals draw in and up in opposition, abs pushing the last of the air out of your lungs.

2. Then inhale and tuck your tailbone under to start the release of your spine back down to the floor. Articulate your spine as you bring each vertebra to the floor one at a time. Start to exhale when your back is midway down on the floor. When your head reaches the floor, extend your arms back up toward the ceiling in the starting position.

Repeat 5 times.

7. SINGLE-LEG CIRCLES

Set-up Bring your arms down by your side, legs onto the floor. Bend one knee into your chest, placing both hands under your knee to stretch your thigh into your chest. Stabilize both your hip bones and shoulders onto the floor, and take a moment to anchor your extended leg still on the floor: Plug the heel of your extended leg onto the floor and reach the ball of your foot away from your hip. Try to draw your shin and back of your thigh down to the floor, thereby stretching your hamstrings and providing a stable base. Turn the top of your extended leg's thigh inward to open up the back of your hip.

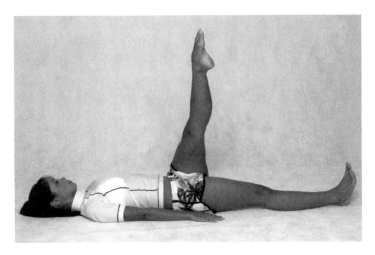

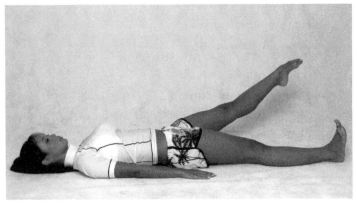

Action

1. Extend the bent leg straight up to the ceiling at 90 degrees to your body and place your hands, palms down, onto the floor. Anchor the lifted leg down into your hip socket and draw that hip away from your ribs. Inhale and cross the lifted leg over the thigh on the floor.

2. Draw your leg down, out, and up to make a circle, exhaling as you lift your leg back up to the start position, at 90 degrees to your body. Inhale for the first half of the circle, exhale for the second half. On each exhalation, scoop your belly in and up. Keep both shoulders and hips still and stabilized on the floor.

Repeat 5 times, then reverse the direction for 5. When done with all 10 repetitions, lower the leg down to the floor, then bend the other knee into your chest before lifting it into the 90-degree position to repeat the exercise on the other side.

Safety Note: *If your back arches or hips lift off the floor when working your legs in a supine position, reduce the range of motion to the point at which you can control the movement while stabilized.*

8. ROLLING LIKE A BALL (Rocking Up to Standing)

Set-up Rock yourself up from the supine position to a seated position on the floor. Place your hands on the floor by your hips, then lift your hips up an inch off the floor, bending at your knees to scoot your seat closer to your heels. Bring your hands around the outside of your legs, to rest on your ankles.

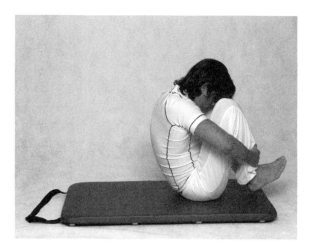 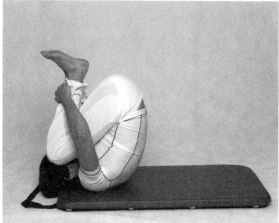

Action

1. Draw your upper body forward and over your abdominals so as to produce a ball-like posture. Elbows should be out wide and to the sides; ears should be between the knees as much as possible, with your shoulders drawn on the back. Scoop into your abdominals and tuck your tailbone under to lift your feet—together with the toes facing down—one inch off the floor. Find your balance.

2. Inhale and draw your abdominals in and up to roll back to the base of your shoulder blades. As you roll back, lift your hips up and dig your heels toward the buttocks. Don't fling your feet up to create momentum! As soon as you've rocked back to your shoulder blades, exhale and dive your head forward between your knees to rock yourself back up to your starting position.

Repeat 8 times. On the 8th repetition, in the rock-back position, cross your arms and legs, exhale, draw up your abdominals, and rock forward to come to a standing position without using your hands.

9. GINGA COM NEGATIVA E ROLÊ (Swinging into Low Crouch and Roll)

Set-up As before, plant your feet hip-width apart and parallel. Keep your knees bent and the weight of your body centered through the balls of your feet.

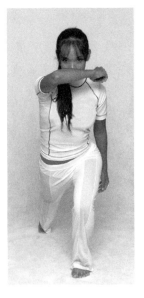 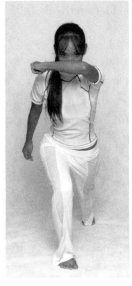

Action

1. Face forward and extend your right leg behind you, pressing back onto the ball of your right foot. Bend your left knee in a slight lunge, keeping the top of your left knee over your left second toe for maximum stability. Raise your right arm up to defend your face as you swing your left arm behind you for balance.

2. Continue to ginga, bringing your right leg forward to come parallel to your left leg and then extending your left leg back as you lunge on your right knee, pressing onto the ball of your left foot. The arm that goes up to defend your face is on the same side as the leg extended behind. As always in the Ginga, keep the center of gravity low by engaging your abdominals, leaning your upper body forward, and tucking your pelvis under as if you were about to sit down.

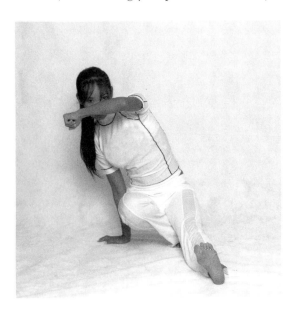

3. For the Negativa, start with your right leg extended behind and your left leg bent in front in a lunge. Sit back almost completely down on your right heel as you extend your left leg in front and bring your right hand to the floor and close in to your right hip. Your left hand should still be up in front of your face in defense. Lean your upper body into your right side and keep your abdominals drawn upward so that you don't collapse over your thighs. Once in position, turn the toes of your extended leg out (in a *roda* when sparring, if the toes still face up, you could get your foot broken!).

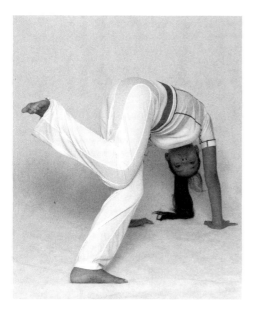

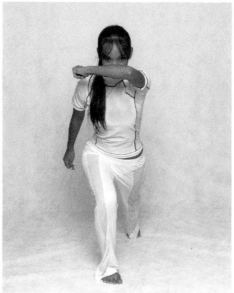

4. Exit the Negativa with a Rolê: Cross your right leg over your extended left leg and bring your hand down to the floor. Lift your hips up. You should now have both hands and feet on the floor, so that you can peek through your legs.

5. Rotate your body further to the right to face forward and swing your left leg so that it will be the leg extended behind and your right knee will be the lunging leg forward. Your left arm comes off the floor to defend your face as your right arm swings back. Continue to ginga.

Repeat 10 full times, alternating between 10 Negativa-Rolês from left-to-right and 10 Negativa-Rolês from right-to-left. Ginga completely on both sides before each Negativa-Rolê.

10. SINGLE-LEG STRETCH

Set-up Center yourself in an upright position, cross your arms and legs, and lower yourself back to a supine position on the floor as before.

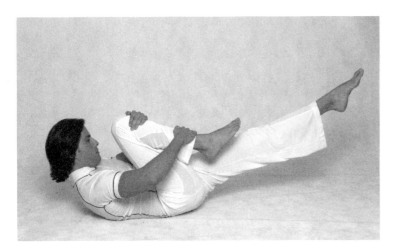

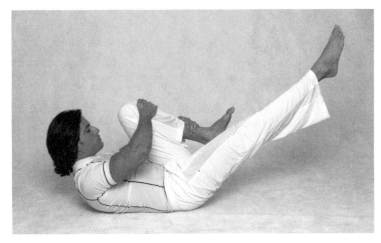

Action

1. Bring your right knee in toward your chest, placing your right hand on your right ankle and your left hand just below your right knee. Extend your elbows out wide to the sides. Draw your chin into your chest by lifting your shoulders up and forward off the floor. Keep the base of your shoulder blades anchored. Extend your left leg out at 45 degrees.

2. Switch legs, reversing your hand placement. Move smoothly as you switch the hands and legs, inhaling for 2 leg switches, then exhaling for 2. Don't tuck your pelvis, sway your hips from side to side, or shift your head. Keep your upper arms lifted.

Repeat 8 times for each leg.

Safety Note: *The Single-Leg Stretch and the following four exercises require your shoulders lifted and chin toward the chest while on your back. If you cannot maintain this through the series, keep your head on the floor.*

11. DOUBLE-LEG STRETCH

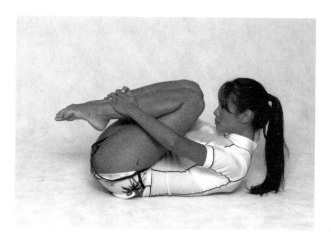

Set-up Bend your knees in toward your chest, hands just above your ankles. Keep your head and neck lifted as you did in the previous exercise, maintaining the base of your shoulder blades rooted to the floor.

Action

Inhale and stretch out, extending your arms and legs away from each other at around 60 degrees. Keep your legs zippered together and your feet soft; make sure your arms are plugged fully back into your shoulders, with your shoulders on the back. Draw your abdominals in and up even more deeply, then exhale as you sweep your arms in a circle to rest above your ankles as your knees draw back into the starting position. Keep your tailbone down at all times.

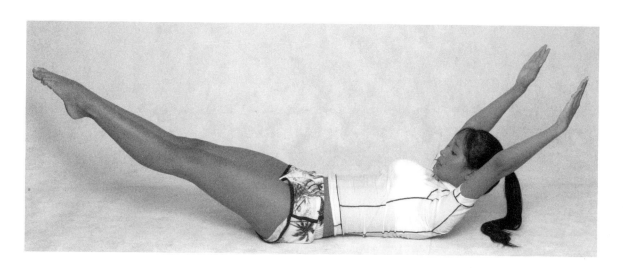

Repeat 8 times.

12. SINGLE STRAIGHT-LEG STRETCH (The Scissors)

Set-up Try to transition directly from the previous exercise into this one. Remain on your back with your abdominals drawn in and up, your shoulders lifted up and forward so that your chin reaches toward your chest. Maintain your gaze on your belly button. Extend both legs up toward the ceiling, and then both arms, forming a U shape with your body.

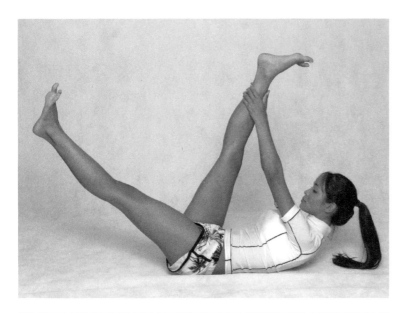

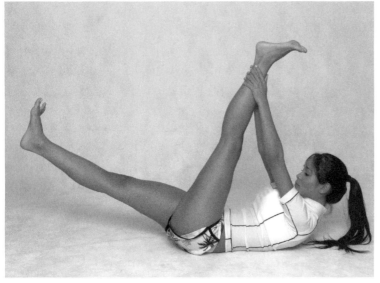

Action

1. With flexed feet, draw your right leg in toward your chest and reach for your ankle with both hands as you double-pulse the leg in. Your left leg scissors down in the opposite direction.

2. Switch legs, now reaching for your left ankle with both hands as your right leg scissors down. Keep the movement vigorous, inhaling for 2 counts, then exhaling for 2 counts. Elbows remain wide to the sides. Both hips and the base of your shoulder blades must stay anchored into the floor, with no wobbling in your head or upper body.

Repeat 8 times for each leg.

13. DOUBLE STRAIGHT-LEG STRETCH (The Lower-Lift)

Set-up As before, try to transition directly from the previous exercise into this one.

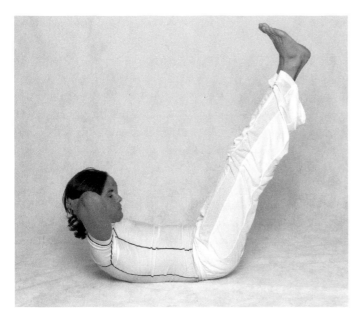

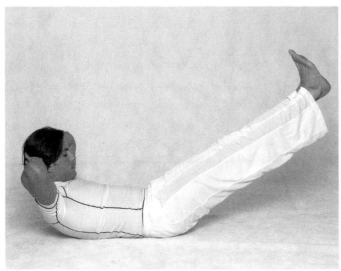

Action

1. Draw both legs together and up toward the ceiling at just below a 90-degree angle to your lower body. Root your tailbone into the floor. Place both hands behind your head, chin tuck into the chest, with shoulders lifted and elbows out wide to the sides. Fix your gaze on your abdominals, keeping them drawn in and up.

2. Inhale and lower your legs in 3 counts toward the floor, to 45 degrees. Draw your abdominals in and up even deeper, then exhale and lift your legs back to the starting position at just below 90 degrees. Press the back of your skull into your hands to draw the energy of your upper body away and in opposition to the energy of your legs' lowering and lifting. If your back arches when your lower your legs, reduce the range of motion by lowering your legs only to about 60 degrees.

Repeat 8 times.

14. CRISS-CROSS

Set-up As before, try to transition directly from the previous exercise into this one. Remain on your back with shoulders lifted, chin toward your chest, and hands behind your head; draw your knees into your chest.

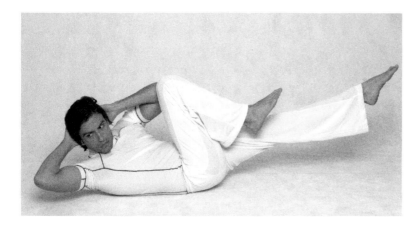

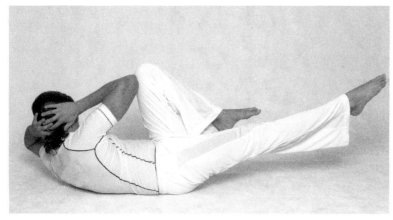

Action

1. Inhale and reach your left elbow to your right knee, extending your left leg out to about 45 degrees.

2. Exhale and bring your right elbow to your left knee, reversing the position and extending the opposite leg. Keep the action rhythmic without snapping your knees or swaying your pelvis. Look over your shoulder as you twist, keeping your elbows out wide to the sides and your shoulders lifted off the floor. Root your hips and the base of your shoulder blades into the floor with your abdominals to stabilize your body as it twists.

Repeat 8 times. When finished, relax your head down to the floor, bend your knees into your chest, and give yourself a quick stretch before crossing your arms and legs and rocking up to a standing position.

15. SPINE-STRETCH FORWARD

Set-up Center yourself in an upright position, your feet hip-width apart and parallel. To lower yourself down from a vertical to a horizontal position as before, cross your arms genie-style, keeping your shoulders on your back and lifting your abdominals in and up, and cross one leg over the other and lower down to the floor without sticking your buttocks out.

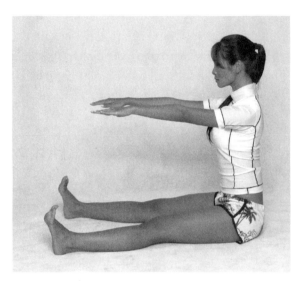 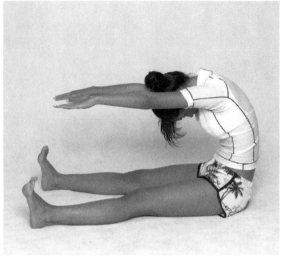

Action

1. When seated, extend your legs out on the floor in front of you and sit up tall. Open your legs so that they are hip-width apart, keeping your feet flexed. Draw yourself up as tall as possible using your abdominals, and extend your arms forward at shoulder height.

2. Inhale and drop your chin into your chest, rounding your back and drawing the crown of your head toward the floor. Keep your arms at shoulder-height and exhale as you reach the arms forward; draw your abdominals up and back in opposition.

Inhale and start to articulate your spine upward. Stack the vertebra one at a time to draw yourself up tall to the starting position, exhaling at the finish.

Repeat 3 times.

16. MODIFIED OPEN-LEG ROCKER

Set-up Place your hands under your thighs and walk your buttocks forward so that your knees bend to an acute angle.

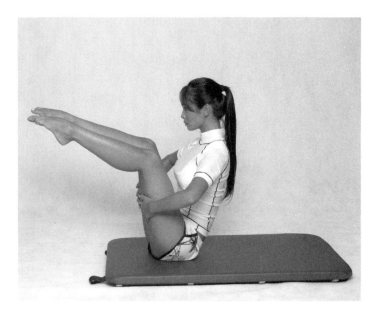

Action

1. Draw your abdominals in and up and lean back to lift your shins up and parallel to the floor. Your legs should still be hip-width apart as they were in the previous exercise. Keep your elbows wide to the sides and your shoulders on your back, using the muscles of your back and sides of the body to lift your waist.

2. Inhale as you drop your chin into the chest and round your back. Rock to the base of your shoulder blades, then exhale and lift your waist to rock up to the starting position. Your shins should remain parallel and hip-width apart. Don't fling your legs overhead as you rock back, and make sure to lift your head after you lift your waist when rocking up.

Repeat 5 times.

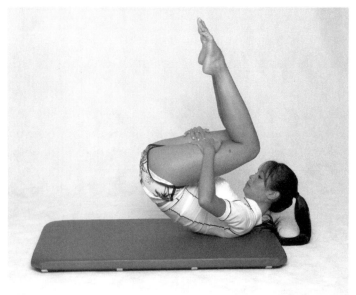

VARIATION: OPEN-LEG ROCKER

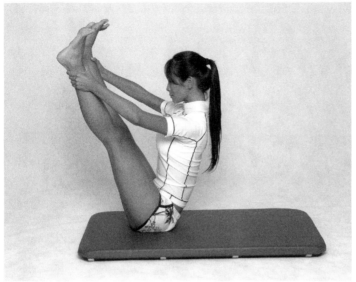

1. For more of a challenge, reach your hands to your ankles and balance on your tailbone with your legs hip-width apart and upward in a V shape. Attempt this only when you have sufficient strength and flexibility to hold your hands on your ankles without bending your knees or opening your legs wider than hip-width apart.

2. Rock back and forth as before in the modified version, and maintain the V shape without bending your legs or shifting your hands.

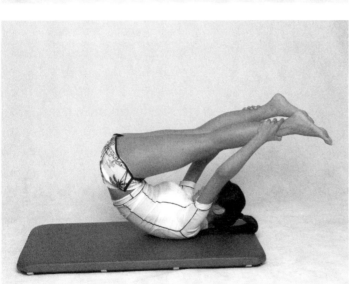

17. CORKSCREW

Set-up Try the following transition from the previous exercise: Close your legs together while still balancing on your tailbone and reach your arms up to a high diagonal. Keep reaching forward with your arms and don't move your legs as you scoop your abdominals and roll your spine down to the floor, one bone at a time.

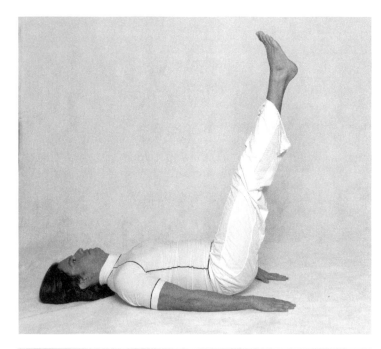

Action

1. When your head touches down, bring your arms by your sides, palms down, and draw your legs together and up toward the ceiling at just below a 90-degree angle. Root your tailbone and shoulders into the floor.

2. Using your lower abdominals, lift your hips vertically off the floor a few inches, then sweep your legs 45 degrees to the right, circle them down, lift them 45 degrees to the left, then lift your hips again once your legs return to the starting position at 90 degrees. Inhale as you start the circle, exhale for the second half of the circle.

Repeat 3 times clockwise, then 3 times counterclockwise.

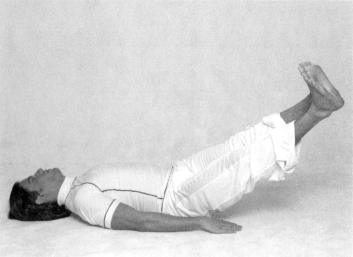

18. THE SAW

Set-up Try the following transition from the previous exercise: Lying down with your legs raised 90 degrees to your upper body, slowly lower both legs down while keeping your shoulders and hips anchored, and your abdominals drawn in and up. Once your legs reach the floor, draw your arms up toward the ceiling, lift your head through your arms, and peel your back off the mat one bone at a time, rising to a seated position.

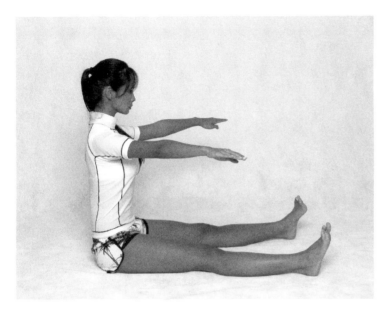

Action

1. Open your legs hip-width apart, flex your feet, and open your arms to the side at shoulder-height.

2. Inhale and twist your waist against your spine to the right. Reach the pinkie of your left hand past your right toe, exhaling as your right arm sweeps back and down like a saw blade. As you reach, draw your left hip down and back, drop your head, and draw your abdominals in and up.

3. Inhale as you lift back to the starting position at center, then twist to the left and reach your right pinkie past your left toe as you exhale. Draw your right hip down and back to stretch.

Repeat 5 times on each side. After 5 repetitions, cross your arms and legs and try lifting to an upright position without using the hands.

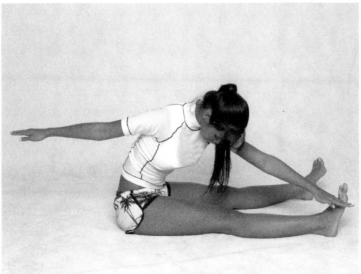

19. SWAN PREP

Set-up Center yourself in an upright position, cross your arms and legs, and lower yourself back to the floor. Swivel your legs behind you, to lie on your belly.

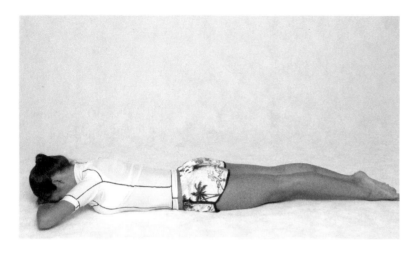

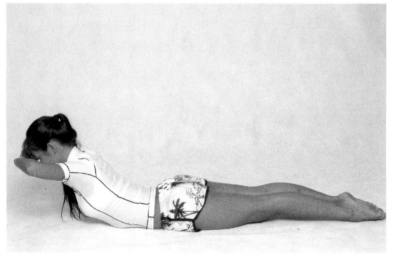

Action

1. Stacking one hand on top of the other, place your hands on the floor and rest your forehead on top of your hands, elbows out to the sides. Anchor your pubic bone into the mat and press your hips and legs into the floor, keeping your feet about six to eight inches apart. Draw the abdominals in and up, making a small space between your belly and the floor.

2. Inhale and lift your upper body, extending it away from your hips while drawing your shoulders on the back. Exhale while lowering back down to the floor. With each successive lift, raise yourself higher, aiming to clear your ribs off the floor. Keep the neck long on the spine.

Repeat 5 times.

20. SINGLE-LEG KICK

Set-up With your chest and abdominals off the floor, place your elbows directly under your shoulders, forearms at 90 degrees to your upper arms. Make a fist with your right hand and close your left hand around it. Draw your legs together, keeping your thighs active and engaged. Don't let your belly droop; keep your abdominals scooped in and up, and anchor your pubic and hip bones into the floor. Draw your shoulders away from your ears and keep your neck long.

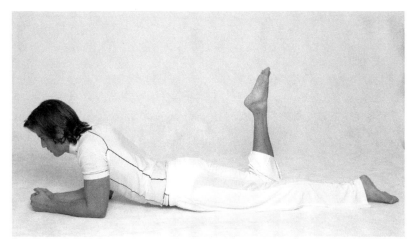

Action

1. Kick your right heel twice into your buttocks.

2. Switch and kick your left heel twice into your buttocks. Move fluidly, and keep your knees from coming apart by engaging your thighs and hamstrings.

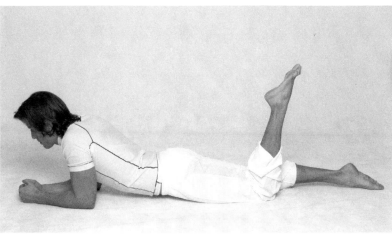

Repeat 5 times on each leg.

21. DOUBLE-LEG KICK

Set-up Bring your head down and your right cheek to the floor. Clasp your hands behind your back between your shoulder blades and draw your elbows toward the floor. Your legs should remain together and active. Keep your abdominals drawn in and upward.

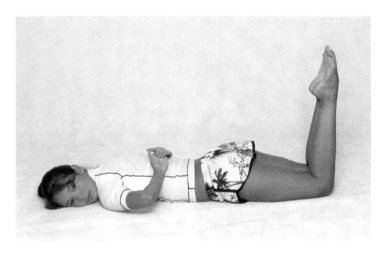

Action

1. Inhale to prepare; then exhale and kick both heels in toward the buttocks three times.

2. Press your hips, legs, and toes into the floor, inhale, and extend your clasped hands as far back as possible while lifting your upper body off the floor. Do not let your legs separate or your toes lift from the floor! Return your head to the floor, this time with your left cheek down.

Repeat 3 times on each side, alternating between each cheek.

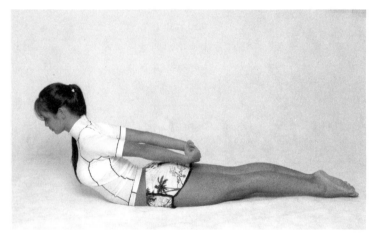

Rest Roll back into a rest position: Sit your hips toward your heels, extending your arms in front of your knees. Keep your knees hip-width apart and feet together. Press the heels of your hands into the floor as you round your back, drop your head down, and pull your abdominals in and up as you stretch your lower back.

22. NECK-PULL WITH AROUND THE WORLD

Set-up Swivel your legs out from under you, extending them to the front as you sit up tall. Open your legs hip-width apart and flex your feet. Place your hands behind your head and press the back of your skull into your hands as you draw yourself to your tallest height. Keep your abdominals scooped in and up.

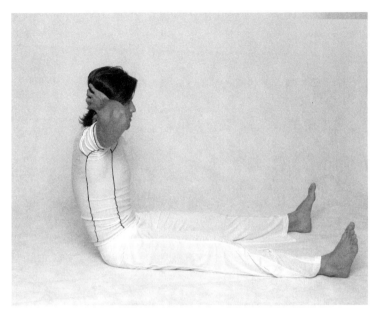

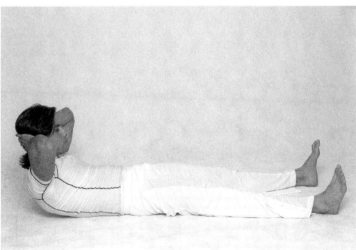

Action

1. Inhale and tuck your tailbone under to start rolling your spine down to the floor, one vertebra at a time. Exhale at the midway point and press the last of the air out of your lungs by the time your head touches down.

2. Take a deep breath in to prepare, then exhale and start to round your spine up and over, bringing your nose between your knees. As you roll up your spine, keep your elbows wide and do not jerk yourself forward to lift; reach the heels of your feet away from the hips and engage your abdominals to maintain control over the articulation!

3. Inhale, stacking your vertebrae up on top of each other as you lift yourself tall to the starting position. Exhale, and this time keep the spine lifted as you hinge back straight from the hip to a 45-degree angle; then tuck your tailbone under and roll your spine back to the floor as you finish exhaling.

Repeat 3 times.

Variation After 3 repetitions, add the following variation: In the upright position, twist your waist against your spine to the right, keeping your elbows wide. Inhale as you lower your back on the right side midway to the floor. Hold your breath as you twist yourself to a center position, keeping your gaze focused on your drawn-in abdominals. Exhale as you twist your waist to the left side and lift yourself up, then twist to finish at the starting position, facing forward.

Repeat 3 times clockwise, and 3 times counterclockwise, alternating the direction after each repetition.

23. SHOULDER-BRIDGE

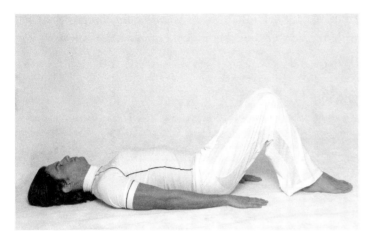

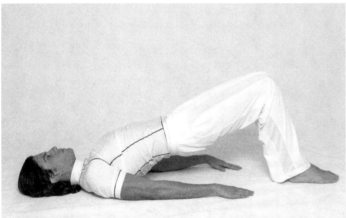

Set-up Lie on your back with your knees bent and the soles of your feet flat on the floor. Keep your feet together and close to your buttocks. Your arms should remain by your side with the palms pressing downward into the floor. Anchor your shoulders and hips as you draw your abdominals in and up.

Action

Inhale to prepare, then exhale, curling your tailbone under and lifting your pelvis upward to form a shoulder-bridge. Keep your knees and thighs together and active, especially while lifted. Inhale to prepare, then exhale and articulate your spine as you lower your back to the floor— dropping first the back of your ribs, then the back of your belly, and finally your tailbone.

Repeat 3 times.

Variation After 3 repetitions, try the following variation: Return to the shoulder-bridge position. Extend your right leg out to 45 degrees, reaching your heel away from your hip. Pulse the leg upward twice toward the ceiling at 90 degrees while keeping both hips at the same level, then flex your foot as you lower it back to 45 degrees. Repeat 3 times on the same leg without dropping your pelvis; after the third repetition, bring your knees together and return the foot to the floor. Your pelvis should still be up in a shoulder-bridge. Exhale as you articulate and lower your spine back to the starting position. Lift back up into a shoulder-bridge and repeat with the other leg 3 times.

24. SIDE SERIES—SIDE KICKS

(This and the following two exercises—Hip Circles and Leg Lifts—are a series. Do the complete series, working one leg, then turn on your other side to switch legs and complete the series again.)

Set-up Lie on your side with your hips and shoulders stacked, your head resting in your hand with your elbow bent, and your upper hand resting on the floor about six to eight inches away from your breastbone. Move your legs out to a 45-degree angle from your upper body.

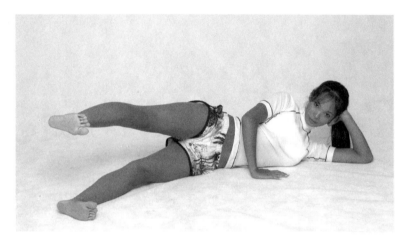

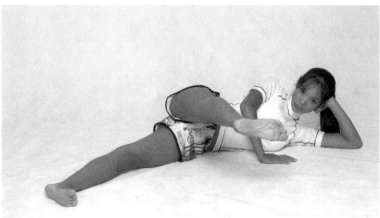

Action

1. Keeping your legs parallel and feet flexed, turn your upper thighs slightly inward toward each other. Lift the upper leg to the height of your hip.

2. Initiating from your lower abdominals, kick your toes with your foot flexed, in the direction of your nose for a double-pulse. Then point the foot and sweep the leg all the way behind you, lifting your abdominals and preventing your upper body from seesawing.

Repeat 6 times.

25. SIDE SERIES—HIP CIRCLES

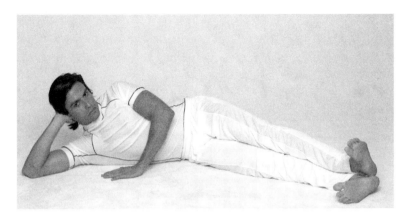

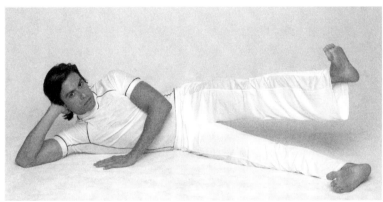

Set-up Remain on your side with your hips and shoulders stacked, your head resting in your hand with your elbow bent, and your upper hand resting on the floor about six to eight inches away from your breastbone. Your legs are still out at a 45-degree angle to your upper body. Rotate your upper leg outward so that the heels of your feet remain connected but the toes of the upper foot extend toward the ceiling.

Action

Circle your upper leg around, brushing the heel of your upper foot past the heel of your lower foot. Reach long through your top leg as you circle it, keeping your abdominals drawn in so that your waist lifts slightly off the mat. Stabilize through your hips so that your upper body does not sway or wobble.

Repeat 5 times.

26. SIDE SERIES—LEG LIFTS

Set-up Remain on your side with your hips and shoulders stacked, your head resting in your hand with your elbow bent, and your upper hand resting on the floor about six to eight inches away from the breastbone. Your legs are still out at a 45-degree angle to your upper body. Keeping your legs parallel, and feet flexed, turn your thighs slightly inward toward each other.

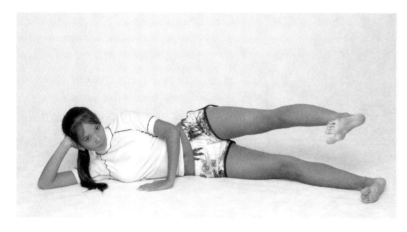

Action

1. Initiating from your abdominals, lift your upper leg—with the foot flexed—in three counts, raising it no higher than a few inches above the hipline.

2. Point the foot and resist as you push the leg back down to the starting position. Perform 10 repetitions, and then reverse the order for 10, lifting the leg with foot pointed and resisting downward with the foot flexed.

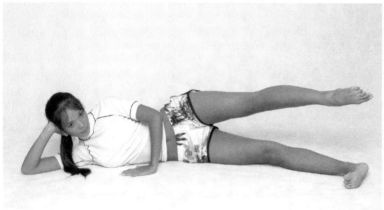

Complete this set, then turn on to your other side and repeat the entire Side Series, starting with the Side Kicks, followed by the Hip Circles, and concluding with the Leg Lifts.

27. GINGA COM BÊNÇÃO (Swinging with "Blessing" Kick)

Set-up When you have completed the Side Series on both sides, roll onto your back, cross your arms and legs, and rock up to a standing position (try not to use your hands if you can). Begin to ginga.

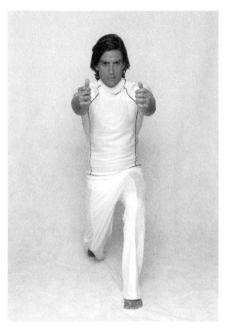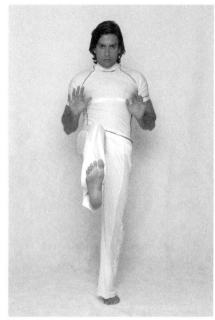

Action

1. As before in the Ginga, face forward and extend your right leg behind you, pressing back onto the ball of your right foot. Bend your left knee in a slight lunge, keeping the top of your left knee over your left second toe for maximum stability. Raise your right arm up to defend your face as you swing your left arm behind you for balance.

2. Step your right foot forward and bend your right knee up as you scoop into your abdominals. Lean and draw your arms forward, almost as if you were about to grab someone by the lapels.

3. Extend your right leg forward into a pushing kick as you lean your upper body back and draw your arms back, elbows bent behind you.

4. Bring your right leg back into the Ginga, and ginga completely on both sides before attempting the kick on the left side.

Repeat 5 times on each side.

28. TEASER

Set-up Center yourself in an upright position, cross your arms and legs, and lower yourself back to a supine position on the floor as before.

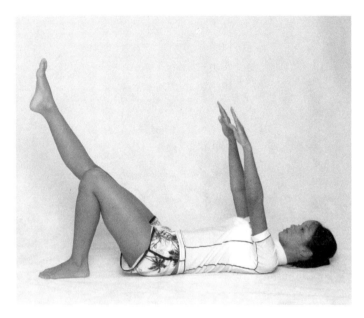

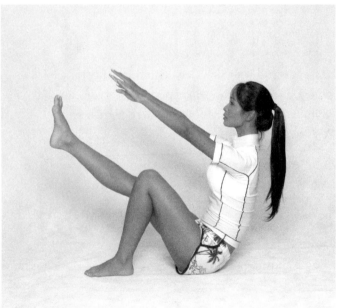

Action

1. Bend your knees and keep the soles of your feet flat on the floor. Press your knees and thighs together and extend one leg out at a 45-degree angle. Anchor your hips and shoulders, and raise your arms toward the ceiling. Keep your shoulders on your back and draw your abdominals in and up.

2. Inhale as you round your back midway off the floor to reach for your knees. Don't jerk your body off the floor or use momentum; move with control and precision.

3. Exhale and reach your hands up to the high diagonal past the toes of your outstretched leg. Keep your foot on the floor firmly planted. Continue to reach for the high diagonal as you inhale, tuck your tailbone under, and roll your back midway to the floor; then exhale and lower all the way back, bringing your arms back to the ceiling in the starting position.

Repeat 3 times.

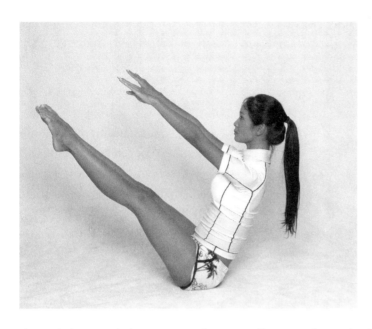

Variation

1. After 3 repetitions, try the following variation: Lie on your back in a "tabletop" position, bending your knees up and over your hips with your shins parallel to the floor. Anchor your hips and shoulders, and raise your arms toward the ceiling. Keep your shoulders on your back and draw your abdominals in and up.

2. Inhale and extend your legs out to a 45-degree angle as you roll your spine upward to reach the hands to the toes. Try to keep your toes at eye-level height and your hands above the sightline. Exhale as you tuck your tailbone under and roll your spine down to the starting position while you continue to reach your arms up in opposition.

Repeat 3 times.

29. SWIMMING

Set-up Lie prone on your belly with your forehead resting on the floor. Your arms and legs should be extended, all limbs hip-width apart. Draw your abdominals in and up, making a bit of space between the floor and your belly.

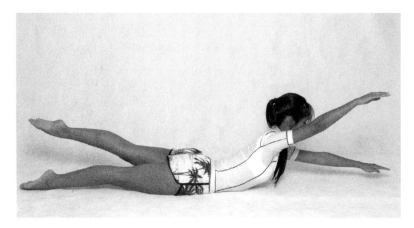

Action

1. Maintain the abdominal engagement as you lift your right arm and your left leg into the air. Keep them there as you lift the other arm and leg. With all four limbs suspended, lift your head off the floor, keeping the neck long.

2. "Swim" by raising and lowering the straight legs and arms rapidly in an alternating fashion for 30 counts. Do not bend the limbs! As you swim, reach your arms long while keeping your shoulders on the back; draw your legs away from your hips, keeping your thighs off the floor.

Rest After 30 counts, roll back into the rest position as before: Sit your hips toward your heels, extending your arms in front of your knees. Keep your knees hip-width apart and your feet together. Press the heels of your hands into the floor as you round your back, drop your head down, and pull your abdominals in and up as you stretch your lower back.

30. SEAL

Set-up Swivel your legs out in front of you as you sit up. Bend your knees to bring your heels together, but keep your knees apart.

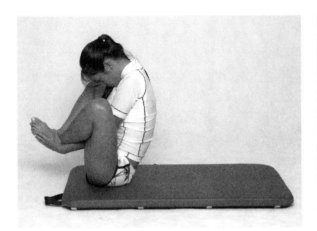
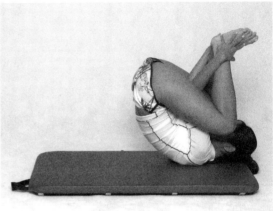

Action

1. Dive your hands through your legs to come up around the outside of your ankles. Round your upper body forward and balance just behind your tailbone as you lift your feet an inch off the floor. Keep your head down and press your forearms in opposition against your thighs. Draw your abdominals in and up, and keep your shoulders on your back.

2. Inhale as you clap your feet twice, then roll back to the base of your shoulder blades. Clap your feet twice again as you lift your hips, then exhale to dive forward to the starting position. Do not drop your feet onto the floor, and resist rolling onto your head and neck.
Repeat 6 times. After you've clapped twice in the roll-back of the sixth repetition, cross your arms and legs, and try to lift yourself to a standing position without using your hands. Pull up into your abdominals and exhale to assist the lift.

When you do the One-Hour Workout and go back to exercises 2, 3, and 4: Ginga com Esquiva pra Trás, Esquiva de Frente, and Esquiva Lateral (Swinging to Dodge from the Rear, from the Front, and from the Side), repeat 30 times on each side, performing the three esquivas ten times each on each side with a complete ginga in between each esquiva. Move as fluidly and rhythmically as possible.

31. ROLL-DOWN WITH PLANK PUSH-UPS

Set-up Center yourself in an upright position. Place your feet parallel, hip-width apart. Lift your abdominals in and up as you draw your shoulders on your back.

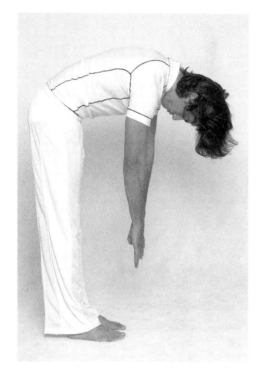

Action

1. Inhale and drop your chin into your chest as you begin rolling your spine down and forward; your abs will lift in and up in opposition. Let your arms, head, and shoulders hang heavy as you unroll your spine and lower your hands all the way to the floor.

2. When your hands reach the floor, walk them out to bring the body into a plank position. Make sure your hands are directly under your shoulders, fingers spread wide apart, abdominals engaged. Bend your elbows behind you for 5 push-ups to the floor. After the fifth push-up, lift your hips toward the ceiling and plant your heels into the floor. Walk your hands back up to your feet without shifting your hips side to side (avoid this by lifting your abs up and rooting your heels into the floor away from your hips). Then roll your spine back up to the standing starting position, one vertebra at a time.

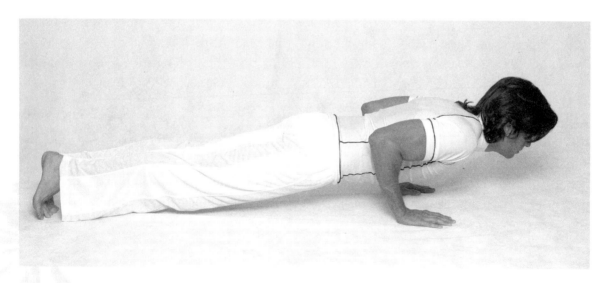

32. BALANCE FINISH

Set-up Rise to the balls of your feet, arms down by your side. Draw your abdominals in and up and keep your shoulders on your back.

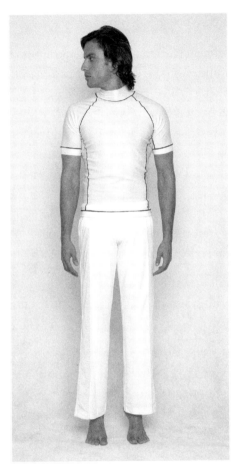 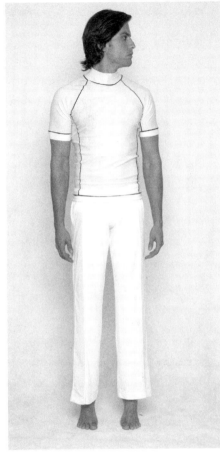

Action

1. Stay still and lifted on the balls of your feet as you turn your head to the right.

2. Turn your head to the left while keeping your balance. Turn your head to center. Lower your heels but try not to lose height in your upper body; lift taller up through your abdominals and ribs as you return to the starting position.

Repeat 3 times.

Jeitinhos for Exercise

"My life is too scattered. Finding time for a workout in between my commitments is too difficult, and by the end of the day I'm too exhausted."

Jeitinho: Set a schedule. If you don't have an electronic organizer, get one. If you can't afford one, buy a pocket-size paperback mini-agenda. People who complain about being pulled in too many directions often do not have detailed time guidelines setting distinct periods aside for all their daily activities. Depending upon where you are in the program, take ten minutes each weekend to consider the week ahead and map out work routines around other activities, placing as much weight on workout time as you would on meals, time with family, social outings, and work. Be realistic about what you can accomplish given how many hours you need to work, but pencil in at least a ten-minute quickie workout each day—to be done either immediately after you awake or three hours before bed—if you can't manage longer sessions during the course of the week. Use the BBBP monthly schedule to figure out your workouts during each day.

"I travel all the time and work exhausting hours on the road. How can I keep up a workout schedule?"

Jeitinho: I used to have this problem myself. My solution was to do three really small workouts (go to the Mini Workout on page 183) each day: in the morning after waking up, at lunchtime in a hotel gym or hotel room, and once again a few hours before going to bed. Breaking up the activity into three small segments made it feel as if it didn't take up quite as much time as if I had taken a half hour out of my schedule. Additionally, I walked everywhere or took public transport. I don't drive, so that part was easy. In general, before I travel, I try to find out if the hotel or neighborhood I'm staying in has a local gym. I always pack a jump rope in my bag—saves on weight and space—so that if I can't find a gym with a day rate, I head out early in the morning to a local park and jump rope for fifteen minutes. Do that every day on the road and your energy levels will increase to the point at which you'll crave the release of working out.

"My house is the size of a shoebox. I don't have enough space to do workouts at home."

Jeitinho: Even if you were living in a prison cell, you'd still have enough room to work out. Rethink how much space you really need. The BBBP workouts are designed to be done in small areas, usually no larger than the length and width of your body. It's a good challenge to try to confine your movements to a certain area. The control necessary to precisely rein in your movements requires more strength and stability. So you actually wind up working a little harder, which is no bad thing. Make sure you have a thick fitness mat to cushion your back. (A plain old yoga mat is NOT sufficient. Be sure to purchase a Pilates mat.)

"I've been doing these exercises for a few weeks and I'm bored. How can I stick with the program?"

Jeitinho: Some people simply need greater motivation to exercise effectively. Working in a group or one-on-one with a teacher might be a better option for people who hit a wall when working out by themselves. Go online to see where you can find capoeira *rodas* in your local area. The interest in capoeira has grown so much that most major cities have at least one capoeira instruction class somewhere. If you can find one, go and experience what it is to actually spar in a capoeira *roda*. It certainly won't be boring! Tradition dictates that in a *roda,* everyone must go into the circle and spar at least once, even if it's your very first time. You might not be able to do very much, but it doesn't matter. People appreciate your effort. You'll also get to sing and perhaps play one of the instruments. When you are "playing" capoeira with others, it makes the idea of physical activity more social. If, however, you do not have the mobility required by capoeira, search for a Pilates equipment-based studio in your area and sign up for a lesson with an instructor. Find a good one in your neighborhood by using the Pilates Method Alliance studio locator (see Resources).

"I've got some injuries. How can I work out?"

Jeitinho: Part of the reason Pilates is such a wonderful exercise is because it's easily modified to accommodate people with injuries. However, if you have considerable rehabilitation issues, you can certainly do Pilates, but you'll need to find an equipment-based studio and an instructor with whom you can work one-on-one. Before you get started, be sure to have a discussion with the instructor about your precise medical or mobility condition. Gradually work your way through your initial sessions. Over time, as your mobility improves, ask your teacher whether it's time to attempt a mat-based workout at home of the kind featured in the BBBP. Continue with a teacher until you can manage some workouts on your own.

"I've been doing the BBBP workouts for a few weeks and I don't see any effects yet. I want to quit!"

Jeitinho: Unfortunately, visible physical changes in the body take time and consistency. Every body reacts differently to the BBBP based on its status before undertaking the program. People with slower metabolisms due to sedentary behavior and poor nutrition will require more time to see visible changes. However, even average people will need to temper their expectations. Despite cover stories in magazines that trumpet hard, six-pack abs in six weeks, the truth is that genetic predisposition and overall conditioning will determine how quickly—and if—you'll develop model middles. Make sure that you give the program thirty days before you make a decision, and follow the workouts daily. Changes may be occurring that you simply can't see. Try this: Each day, stand with your feet hip-width apart, heels down and toes lifted, and with your abdominals lifted in and up. Roll forward by articulating your spine down to the floor. See how far you can get your hands on the floor each day. In the beginning of the BBBP, chances are you won't get down to the floor while keeping your heels down and your toes lifted up. But as the days progress, you'll probably be able to get farther and farther down, a sign of visible progress in your flexibility. Little by little, as your metabolism increases and you burn fat more effectively, you'll see toning around your middle.

"If this is such good exercise, why am I having back pain?"

Jeitinho: Pain is the body's warning signal. If you develop back pain of any kind, stop what you're doing right away. You're probably not engaging your abdominal muscles properly to support the back sufficiently. Another potential problem may be misalignment. As a Pilates instructor, I see this all the time. I ask clients to lie down in what they think is a straight position and about 60 percent of the time, their bodies curve to one side or another. If you work out like this, the misalignment might trigger backache. Find a reputable instructor in your neighborhood and take a few sessions to pinpoint the problem. After locating the problem, see if you can return to the BBBP workouts on your own without experiencing pain. If the pain continues, consult a physician to assess your condition. If given a go-ahead to work out, consider instructor-aided workouts until you become more comfortable with the movements.

"My partner needs to exercise but I can't get him/her motivated. What do I do?"

Jeitinho: First, don't nag or drop what you think are subtle hints. Nobody appreciates being pestered. Have one discussion—calmly, gently, quietly—and then leave off trying to press the matter. From that point onward, plan activities together that can put your partner in a better frame of mind to start working out. Check out Pilates studios or capoeira *rodas* in your neighborhood, and buy a gift package for your partner for encouragement. Plan an active holiday that will allow both of you to try a challenging sport together. Suggest taking hikes or bike rides. A partner who won't do the BBBP workouts may prefer to be active in another way. Don't give up on your partner. In time, if you stay positive and keep providing nonverbal encouragement, your partner might come around. But remember, don't force it—that's the quickest way to destroy any hope for dialogue.

"I can't understand these exercises. They're too complicated."

Jeitinho: The first workouts will always be tricky. You're attempting complex movements that you've never done before and that require exertion. Don't get discouraged. I teach Pilates to professional athletes and their first ten sessions are usually a revelation, humbling them to a level that they've not experienced before. If the workouts were easy, they wouldn't be workouts. Give yourself time to do them right and don't beat yourself up. It's just exercise. If you need extra help, contact a Pilates studio and take one session under the supervision of a teacher. If that doesn't work, consider renting a DVD to see how the movements can be done properly. I recommend the *Classical Pilates Technique: The Complete Mat Workout Series* DVD (see Resources).

"I'm clumsy and have never been athletic. I don't think I can manage these exercises."

Jeitinho: People's perceptions of their own abilities aren't always based in fact. If you grew up being told you were a clumsy child, chances are you still believe that to some degree. You'll need to divest yourself of any negative preconceptions you have before commencing the BBBP. Start with the short workouts first and increase the intensity slowly. Don't waste time worrying about how quickly you get the workouts done. Simply follow the instructions as carefully and as conscientiously as possible. If, after several attempts, you find you need some coaching, consider getting an instructor. If after working with an instructor you find that these exercises just aren't right for you, think about other ways in which you can be active. Consider buying a pedometer, and make walking your activity. Try to rack up more miles each week and add some difficulty to it, like running up a few flights of stairs. Look into other forms of exercise if walking aggravates any medical conditions. In the end, find something you like and do it—just make sure that you elevate the intensity of whatever activity you pursue in order to ensure some benefits. Light exercise, like walking, is simply not enough to make changes in your fitness levels.

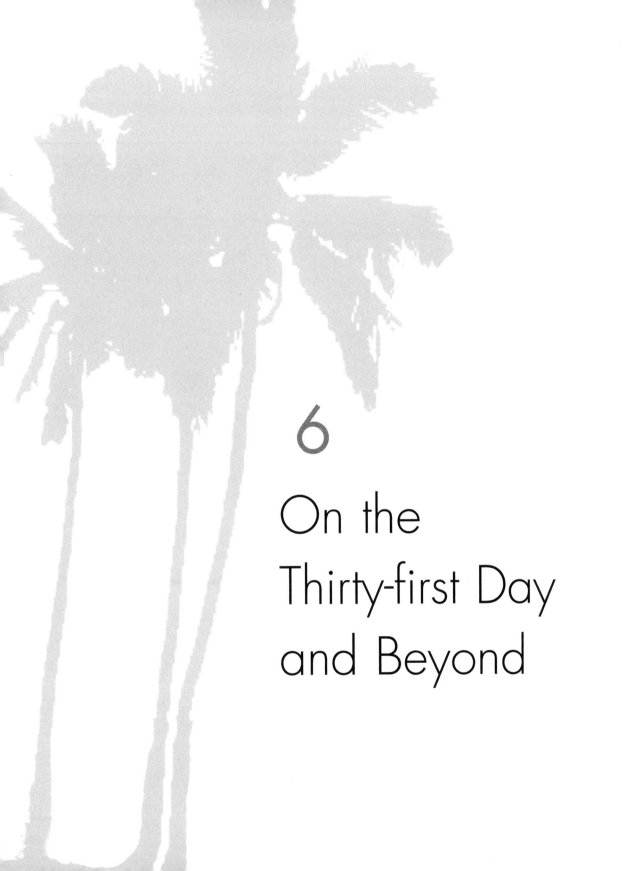

6

On the
Thirty-first Day
and Beyond

The Wrap-up

SO NOW you're on your own. Don't panic!

If you've followed the menus and the workouts pretty closely, well done! Anything that's worth doing takes effort and this lifestyle change does require some work. But after thirty days, you've probably settled into a rhythm in the kitchen, on your workout mat, and in how to improve your quality of life. By this point, you should have experienced an increase in muscle tone, better energy levels, and a greater sense of well-being. If you keep it up, the program's benefits shall continue to accrue—providing you with a happier disposition and perhaps a different outlook on your role in life and the impact you have as an individual on your environment.

Moving forward, consider what was easiest to maintain with respect to both food and movement. To keep up good eating habits, select the recipes you enjoyed the most and found easiest to prepare. Make these your first tier of go-to recipes. This first tier should contain a good balance of healthy superfood ingredients, so try to ensure that each day you consume at least six ingredients from this group:

> Açaí
> Acerola
> Beans, lentils, and chickpeas
> Brazil nuts and cashews
> Kale, spinach, and watercress
> Fish and shrimp
> Lean meat and chicken
> Garlic and onions
> Tomatoes
> Coconut water/milk
> Maté

For the second tier, mix and match from the remaining recipes, or research new recipes that incorporate the basic Brazilian pantry staple ingredients. Go to www.thebrazilianbikinibodyprogram.com for more recipes and information. Over the course of every week, rotate between your first and second tier selections to maintain the basic principles of the program.

After thirty days of trying out the three main exercise routines and making them part of your daily activities, you should have also established a routine of which work-outs work best on which days and at which times. If you find that, after thirty days, you still struggle with making the workouts part of your daily schedule, take a moment to identify what type of sports or movements you love. Then, use this time to determine how to add these movements to your life on a daily basis. Remember, getting this right is a lifelong process involving trial and error, so be prepared to adjust your choices. De-velop new options. Try out sports you've never experienced and see if you like them. Keep trying new things until you find something that sticks. Try not to fall into old couch potato habits by limiting your hours of television or other screen time to no more than four per day.

Make copies of the menu and workout logs (see page 250). Each week, fill out both your eating and workout habits. Each Sunday when you wake up, have a look to see how your week went. If you notice bad habits creeping in, select one week at random from the thirty-day program and try to follow it as closely as possible. Then go back to trying to construct a weekly schedule on your own. Building confidence in your own abilities to follow the basic ideas behind the Brazilian Bikini Body Program is as much an exercise as anything you'll find in the workouts.

Keeping logs can be a little bit of a chore. Try to avoid laziness while scribbling down your day's activities. But I recognize that we all have our busy periods. So if you find yourself too swamped to log your day's meals and movements, employ a *jeitinho*: If you're like a lot of people, your cell phone probably has a camera function. Each time you have a meal, take a photo of what you're eating. Right after a daily workout, snap a photo. At the end of the week on Sunday, scroll through the images you've taken and see whether or not you've managed to stick to your first- and second-tier choices, as well as your movement plan.

Maybe the foregoing doesn't apply to you. It's possible that after all your attempts in the first thirty days of the program, you had little success in following the plan closely. Instead of allowing yourself to quit or start the downward spiral of guilt and re-crimination over failing to change your lifestyle, at least take another stab at it by log-ging your eating and activity habits. As before, if you find yourself too lazy to scribble things down, at least take photos of what you are eating and drinking and each day's ac-tivity. By week's end, if you don't have at least five activity snapshots, and if you have more than seven snaps featuring you eating a lot of pizza or junk food, processed food, fried food, or drinking soft drinks and giant-size coffee drinks, you need to sit down and consider your future.

Think about what's important to you: your family and friends, your career, your self-esteem. Then think about the effect on all three of those things if your health began to deteriorate. Visualize the beneficial impact of making one new positive addition into your life each week—whether that involves eating a bowl of kale every week, or doing the Mini Workout every day for a week, or whatever small step you think you can achieve. Then do it. Each week thereafter, try to build on that by committing to making one more positive change in the coming week. Triumphs may be small, and change may be slow going, but do not give up. Over time, and it may indeed take a long time, you'll have at least taken active steps to try to preserve your place within those three elements that matter the most to you.

Keep your sense of humor. Do your best. And bear in mind that you have tomorrow to perfect what you couldn't quite get right today. The key is in not giving up and at least making an honest attempt. Employ this gentle *jeito* to what you do, and no matter how you've fared, you'll still be living the Bikini Body Program lifestyle.

Agora vai! Now go!

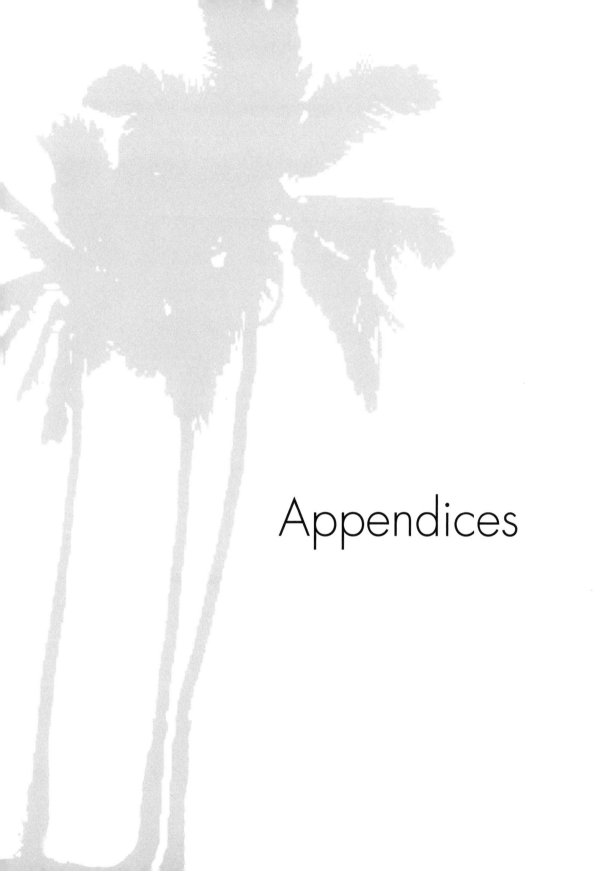

Appendices

WEEK 1 / WEEKLY FOOD PREPARATION CALENDAR

SUNDAY, DAY 1

- Shop for groceries (see Week 1 Shopping List on page 240).
- Dice onions and peppers, and refrigerate in airtight containers for week's use.
- Hard-boil a few eggs and refrigerate in airtight containers for week's use.
- Prepare Garlic Wine Marinade and refrigerate in airtight bottle for week's use (see recipe on page 76).
- Prepare Green Aroma and refrigerate in airtight container for week's use (see recipe on page 77).
- Prepare Limacello if you have time (see recipe on page 75).
- Prepare Coriander-Garlic Sauce and refrigerate in airtight container for week's use (see recipe on page 86).

- Prepare Chickpea Salad and refrigerate in airtight container for week's use (see recipe on page 90).
- Prepare nut recipes and store in airtight containers for month's use (see recipes on pages 103, 104, and 105).
- Prepare Nut-Crusted Apple Pie and refrigerate in airtight container for week's use (see recipe on page 158).
- Prepare a quart of maté tea with lime and refrigerate in an airtight pitcher for this week's use (see recipe on page 69).
- Prepare Empada and Shrimp Empadinhas (see recipes on page 138; Shrimp Empadinhas are to be frozen for later use).

TUESDAY, DAY 3

- Grill enough chicken tonight to have for lunch tomorrow.

- In the evening, marinate steaks in Garlic Wine for dinner tomorrow (see recipe on page 124).

WEDNESDAY, DAY 4

- Prepare Black Bean Salad and store in airtight container for week's use (see recipe on page 91).
- Prepare Fruit Salad (see recipe on page 162).
- Grill enough steak tonight to have for lunch tomorrow.

- If possible, marinate chicken for Chicken Stroganoff for dinner tomorrow in Garlic Wine tonight (see recipe on page 118).

SATURDAY, DAY 7

- Shop for groceries (see Week 2 Shopping List on page 242).
- Dice onions and peppers, and refrigerate in airtight containers for week's use.
- Prepare Garlic Wine Marinade and refrigerate in airtight bottle for week's use (see recipe on page 76).
- Prepare Green Aroma and refrigerate in airtight container for week's use (see recipe on page 77).

- Prepare Coconut Flan and Prune Compote and refrigerate in airtight containers for week's use (see recipes on page 161 and 163).
- Grind ½ cup each of cashews and peanuts to make ground nut powders for following weeks. Store in airtight containers.
- Marinate oxtail tonight in Garlic Wine Marinade for Oxtail and Watercress Stew lunch tomorrow (see recipe on page 126).

WEEK 2

SUNDAY, DAY 8

- Prepare Nutty Mango Vinaigrette and refrigerate in airtight container for week's use (see recipe on page 81).
- Prepare Lentil Salad and refrigerate in airtight container for week's use (see recipe on page 89).
- Hard-boil a few eggs and refrigerate in airtight containers for week's use.
- Prepare Spinach Sauce and refrigerate in airtight container for week's use (see recipe on page 78).

MONDAY, DAY 9

- Marinate pork loin in Garlic Wine tonight for Roasted Pork Loin dinner tomorrow (see recipe on page 117).

TUESDAY, DAY 10

- Make sure to leave enough slices of tonight's Roasted Pork Loin dinner for lunch sandwiches tomorrow.

WEDNESDAY, DAY 11

- Prepare enough turkey for tonight's dinner to have for lunch tomorrow.
- Prepare Brazilian Fudge Balls and refrigerate in airtight container for week's use (see recipe on page 154).

FRIDAY, DAY 13

- Buy fish for dinner tonight and ask the fishmonger for fish head scraps to make Pirão.

SATURDAY, DAY 14

- Shop for groceries (see Week 3 Shopping List on page 244).
- Dice onions and peppers, and refrigerate in airtight containers for week's use.
- Prepare Garlic Wine Marinade and refrigerate in airtight bottle for week's use (see recipe on page 76).
- Prepare Green Aroma and refrigerate in airtight container for week's use (see recipe on page 77).
- If necessary, prepare nut recipes and store in airtight containers for month's use (see recipes on pages 103, 104, and 105).
- Prepare Malted Milk Panna Cottas and refrigerate in airtight containers for week's use (see recipe on page 153).
- Prepare Pirão croutons and freeze for use next week (see recipe for Pirão on page 83 and recipe for croutons on page 94).
- In the evening, marinate meat in Garlic Wine for Cozido lunch tomorrow (see recipe on page 121).

WEEK 3

SUNDAY, DAY 15

- Prepare Coriander-Garlic Sauce and refrigerate in airtight container for week's use (see recipe on page 86).
- Prepare Arugula Sauce and refrigerate in airtight container for week's use (see recipe on page 80).
- Prepare Chunky Vinaigrette and refrigerate in airtight container for week's use (see recipe on page 80).
- Prepare Hijiki Salad and refrigerate in airtight container for week's use (see recipe on page 152).
- Prepare Watercress Soup and refrigerate or freeze in airtight container for week's use (see recipe on page 110).
- Retrieve the Limacello, strain, and mix with sugar syrup before storing again for another week (see recipe on page 75).
- Prepare a quart of maté tea with lime and refrigerate in an airtight pitcher for this week's use (see recipe on page 69).
- Hard-boil a few eggs and refrigerate in airtight containers for next week's use.

MONDAY, DAY 16

- Grill enough chicken for dinner tonight to have for tomorrow's lunch.
- In the evening, marinate steaks in Garlic Wine for dinner tomorrow (see recipe on page 125).

TUESDAY, DAY 17

- Grill enough steak tonight to have for tomorrow's lunch sandwiches.
- Prepare Wobbly Marias and refrigerate in airtight containers for week's use (see recipe on page 159).

WEDNESDAY, DAY 18

- Marinate chicken in Garlic Wine overnight for Frango à Passarinho dinner tomorrow (see recipe on page 141).

THURSDAY, DAY 19

- Take croutons out of freezer and defrost for tomorrow's Eggplant Salad lunch.

FRIDAY, DAY 20

- Buy sushi-grade fish for dinner party this morning or afternoon.

SATURDAY, DAY 21

- Shop for groceries (see Week 4 Shopping List on page 246).
- Dice onions and peppers, and refrigerate in airtight containers for week's use.
- Prepare Garlic Wine Marinade and refrigerate in airtight bottle for week's use (see recipe on page 76).
- Prepare Green Aroma and refrigerate in airtight container for week's use (see recipe on page 77).
- If necessary, grind ½ cup each of cashews and peanuts for use in this week's recipes.
- Prepare Açaí-Strawberry Puddings and refrigerate in airtight containers for week's use (see recipe on page 155).
- Prepare Acarajé and freeze some of the batch for use next week (see recipe on page 100).

WEEK 4

- Prepare Watercress Sauce and refrigerate in airtight container for week's use (see recipe on page 78).
- Prepare Black Bean Soup and refrigerate in airtight container for week's use (see recipe on page 107).
- Prepare Cabbage Salad and refrigerate in airtight container for week's use (see recipe on page 151).
- Prepare a quart of maté tea with lime and refrigerate in an airtight pitcher for this week's use (see recipe on page 69).
- Hard-boil a few eggs and refrigerate in airtight containers for next week's use.
- Retrieve the finished Limacello and make Limacello Vinaigrette (see recipe on page 85). Put the Limacello in a freezer and refrigerate the vinaigrette in an airtight container.

MONDAY, DAY 23

- Make enough Brazilian Mincemeat to use for lunch tomorrow.

TUESDAY, DAY 24

- Make sure to cook enough chicken from the dinner tonight to use for tomorrow's lunch.
- Prepare Coconut-Tapioca Pudding and refrigerate in an airtight container for week's use (see recipe on page 156).
- In the evening, marinate steaks in Garlic Wine for dinner tomorrow (see recipe on page 125).

WEDNESDAY, DAY 25

- Make sure to cook enough steak from the dinner tonight to use for tomorrow's lunch.

FRIDAY, DAY 27

- Buy fish fresh today for tonight's dinner, Vatapá (see recipe on page 129).
- Soak and refrigerate enough salt cod in milk tonight for both tomorrow and Sunday's recipes, Cod Gomes de Sá and Salt Cod Fritters (see recipes on pages 135 and 101).

SATURDAY, DAY 28

- Shop for groceries (see Week 5 Shopping List on page 248).
- Dice onions and peppers, and refrigerate in airtight containers for week's use.
- Cut up fruit required for tomorrow's cocktails and refrigerate in an airtight container (your choice of fruit).
- Prepare Garlic Wine Marinade and refrigerate in airtight bottle for week's use (see recipe on page 76).
- Prepare Green Aroma and refrigerate in airtight container for week's use (see recipe on page 77).
- While cooking potatoes for tonight's dinner, Cod Gomes de Sá, boil several extra cups of potatoes to have for use in tomorrow's Salt Cod Fritters and for the following Monday's Caldo Verde (see recipes on pages 135, 101, and 109). Refrigerate the mashed potatoes in an airtight container.
- Marinate the meats in Garlic Wine for tomorrow's Feijoada (see recipe on page 123).
- Soak dried black beans overnight in water for tomorrow's Feijoada.
- If necessary, grind ½ cup each of cashews and peanuts for use in this week's recipes.
- Prepare Orange Cake and refrigerate in airtight container for week's use (see recipe on page 160).

WEEK 5

- Prepare Pepper Sauce and refrigerate in airtight container for week's use (see recipe on page 82).
- Cut kale in a chiffonade and refrigerate in airtight container for week's use.
- Prepare Cheese Rolls and freeze any leftovers (see recipe on page 99).
- Prepare Salt Cod Fritters and freeze any leftovers (see recipe on page 135).

- Prepare a quart of maté tea with lime and refrigerate in an airtight pitcher for this week's use (see recipe on page 69)
- Hard-boil a few eggs and refrigerate in airtight container for next week's use.
- Marinate chicken in Garlic Wine for tomorrow's dinner, Ximxim de Galinha (see recipe on page 140).

MONDAY, DAY 30

- Look into your refrigerator and pantry, and think about your menus for the next thirty days. Make sure you have enough until the following Saturday when you do the next round of grocery shopping.

Weekly Shopping Lists

TIP: Each list details weekly supplies for a household of up to two people. Increase accordingly to suit the number of household members or people for whom you're cooking. Bear in mind that several items in the Week 1 list may be sufficient to last several weeks for more than one person (e.g, nuts, spices, oils, vinegars, and other condiments). After Week 1, the subsequent weekly shopping lists will have items you need to buy or restock highlighted in bold. Simply check your pantry for the items that have not been highlighted to see if you have enough for the coming week; if you do, cross them off the list.

WEEK 1

- Frozen *açaí* pulp (sweetened and infused with *guaraná*)—2 packages of 4 (3.5-ounce) packets or 2 (1-pint) tubs
- Frozen acerola pulp—1 package of 4 (3.5-ounce) packets
- Frozen strawberries—16-ounce package (or same amount fresh)
- Frozen blueberries—16-ounce package (or same amount fresh)
- Frozen cut mangoes—16-ounce package (or same amount fresh)
- Frozen cut mixed fruit (berries, melon, etc.)—16-ounce package (or same amount fresh)
- Frozen shrimp—2 (16-ounce) packages (or same amount fresh)
- Frozen chicken stock—10-ounce container (or same amount fresh)
- Frozen broccoli—16-ounce package (or same amount fresh)
- Frozen or dried shiitake mushrooms—16-ounce package (or same amount fresh)
- Frozen piecrust—2 (16-ounce) packages
- Coconut water—4 (11-ounce) portions
- Vanilla soy milk—1 quart
- Unflavored soy milk—1 pint
- Buttermilk—1 half gallon
- Reduced-fat sour cream—8-ounce container
- Reduced-fat cream cheese—8-ounce container
- Feta cheese—6-ounce container
- Grated Parmesan—8-ounce container

- Cream (heavy or half-and-half)—1 pint
- Orange juice—1 quart
- 1 dozen eggs

- Bacon (turkey or pork)—1-pound package
- Small red meat fillet (beef, buffalo, or ostrich)—1 pound
- Beef (cut into cubes)—2 pounds
- Whole chicken breast—3 large
- Fish—1 small whole fish (e.g., snapper, trout), cleaned and gutted

- Garlic—3 heads
- Onions—5-pound bag
- Red onion—1
- Scallions—1 bunch
- Carrots—1-pound bag
- Radishes—1 bunch
- Parsley—3 bunches (curly-leaf)
- Coriander—3 bunches
- Romaine lettuce—1 head
- Watercress—3 bunches
- Arugula—1 bunch
- Spinach—1-pound bag
- Celery—1-pound bag
- Cucumber—1
- Beet—1
- Red bell pappers—3
- Green bell peppers—2
- Yellow bell peppers—2

240

- Ginger—1 medium-size knob
- Tomatoes—1 dozen
- Cherry tomatoes—1 pint
- Limes—2 dozen
- Lemons—6
- Oranges—2
- Bananas—6
- Apples—3 green apples, 3 red apples
- Pear—1
- Chickpeas—2 (15-ounce) cans, or 1 (16-ounce) bag dried
- Black beans—2 (15-ounce) cans, or 1 (16-ounce) bag dried
- Roasted nori seaweed (preferably teriyaki or hot-and-spicy flavored, in hand-roll cut size)—.8-ounce package

- Brazil nuts—1 pound
- Cashews—1 pound
- Walnuts—1 pound
- Peanuts—½ pound
- Peanut butter (crunchy or creamy)—16-ounce jar
- Pumpkin seeds—1 pound
- Dates—8-ounce package
- Dried figs—6-ounce pacakge
- Raisins—15-ounce package
- Dried prunes—9-ounce package
- Pressed guava paste or *membrillo*—21-ounce package
- Apple juice—1 quart
- Honey—8-ounce jar

- Palm hearts—3 (14-ounce) cans
- Coconut milk—2 (14-ounce) cans
- Green olives with pimientos—6-ounce jar
- Capers—6-ounce jar
- Artichoke hearts in olive oil—12-ounce jar
- Chipotle peppers in adobo—7-ounce can
- Malagueta peppers—5-ounce jar of preserved peppers, or 2 fresh
- Japanese pickles—7-ounce package

- Extra-virgin olive oil—34-ounce bottle
- *Dendê* oil—7-ounce bottle
- Sesame oil—6-ounce bottle
- Canola oil—32-ounce bottle
- Red wine vinegar—17-ounce bottle
- Balsamic vinegar—17-ounce bottle
- Soy sauce (preferably reduced-sodium) or tamari—15-ounce bottle
- Mirin (Japanese cooking wine)—17-ounce bottle

- Bay leaves—.5-ounce container
- Ground cinnamon—2.4-ounce container
- Ground allspice—2-ounce container
- Ground cloves—2-ounce container
- Ground coriander—1.6-ounce container
- Ground nutmeg—2.4-ounce container
- Ground cumin—3-ounce container
- Dried oregano—1.1-ounce container
- Cayenne—2-ounce container
- Garlic powder—2.4-ounce container
- Black peppercorns—2.4-ounce container

- Tabasco or hot pepper sauce (preferably made with malagueta peppers)—5-ounce bottle
- Whole-grain mustard (preferably Pommery)—12-ounce jar
- Ketchup—24-ounce bottle
- Maté tea—1 box of tea bags
- Brown rice (preferably Texmati or other brown basmati)—2-pound package
- Sugar—2-pound package
- Splenda—1.9-ounce box
- Whole wheat flour—2-pound package
- Cornstarch—16-ounce box
- Whole wheat wraps—1 package of 4–6 wraps

- White wine (Riesling, Gewürztraminer, or Portuguese *vinho verde*)—1 bottle
- *Cachaça* (to prepare Limacello)—1 bottle
- Armagnac or Cognac—1 bottle

- Frozen *açaí* pulp (sweetened and infused with *guaraná*)—2 packages of 4 (3.5-ounce) packets, or 2 1-pint tubs
- Frozen acerola pulp—1 package of 4 (3.5-ounce) packets
- Frozen strawberries—16-ounce package (or same amount fresh)
- Frozen blueberries—16-ounce package (or same amount fresh)
- Frozen cut mangoes—16-ounce package (or same amount fresh)
- Frozen cut mixed fruit (berries, melon, etc.)—16-ounce package
- Frozen shrimp—16-ounce package (or same amount fresh)
- Frozen chicken stock—10-ounce container (or same amount fresh)
- Frozen vegetable stock—10-ounce container (or same amount fresh)
- Frozen beef stock—10-ounce container (or same amount fresh)
- Frozen broccoli—16-ounce package (or same amount fresh)
- Frozen shiitake mushrooms—16-ounce package (or same amount fresh or dried)

- Coconut water—4 (11-ounce) portions
- Vanilla soy milk—1 quart
- Unflavored soy milk—1 pint
- Buttermilk—1 half gallon
- Milk—1 half gallon
- Reduced-fat sour cream—8-ounce container
- Reduced-fat cream cheese—8-ounce container
- Unflavored live yogurt—8-ounce container
- Grated Parmesan cheese—8-ounce container
- Tofu—14-ounce container
- Cream (heavy or half-and-half)—1 pint
- Orange juice—1 quart
- 1 dozen eggs

- Bacon (turkey or pork)—1-pound package
- Pork loin—3 pounds
- Ground beef or lamb, very lean—2 pounds
- Oxtails, trimmed extra-lean—2 pounds
- *Chouriço*—2 sausages
- Whole chicken—2 pounds
- Turkey breast—1
- Fish—2 (8-ounce) whole fish (e.g. sole, catfish, trout), cleaned and gutted
- Dried, smoked shrimp—¼ pound

- Garlic—3 heads
- Onions—5-pound bag
- Red onions—2
- Scallions—1 bunch
- Potatoes—5-pound bag, preferably fingerling or Yukon Gold
- Carrots—1-pound bag
- Radishes—1 bunch
- Fennel—1 bulb
- Cauliflower—1 head
- Parsley—3 bunches
- Coriander—3 bunches
- Mint—1 bunch
- Romaine lettuce—1 head
- Kale—1 large bunch (preferably "black" or Cavolo Nero kale)
- Watercress—5 bunches
- Arugula—1 bunch
- Spinach—1-pound bag
- Celery—1-pound bag
- Cucumber—1
- Yucca—1 large root
- Red bell peppers—3
- Green bell peppers—2
- Yellow bell peppers—2
- Malagueta peppers—2
- Tomatoes—6
- Limes—1 dozen
- Lemons—6
- Oranges—2

- Bananas—6
- Apples—6
- Pears—2
- Chickpeas—2 (15-ounce) cans, or 1 (16-ounce) bag dried
- Black beans—2 (15-ounce) cans, or 1 (16-ounce) bag dried
- Fava beans—2 (15-ounce) cans, or 1 (16-ounce) bag dried
- Lentils—16-ounce bag Puy or small green lentils
- Bulgur wheat—1 (24-ounce) package
- Hon-dashi powder ("dashi-no-moto" or instant miso soup mix)—(10-packet) package
- Roasted nori seaweed (preferably teriyaki or hot-and-spicy flavored)—.8-ounce container

- Brazil nuts—1 pound
- Cashews—1 pound
- Walnuts—1 pound
- Peanuts—½ pound
- Peanut butter (crunchy or creamy)—16-ounce jar
- Pumpkin seeds—1 pound
- Pressed guava paste or *membrillo*—21-ounce package

- Palm hearts—2 (14-ounce) cans
- Coconut milk—3 (14-ounce) cans
- Tuna in spring water—6-ounce can
- Red miso—15-ounce container
- Concentrated tomato paste—12-ounce container
- Horseradish—4-ounce container
- Pitted black gaeta olives—15-ounce container
- Japanese pickles—7-ounce package

- Extra-virgin olive oil—34-ounce bottle
- *Dendê* oil—7-ounce bottle
- Sesame oil—6-ounce bottle
- Canola oil—32-ounce bottle
- Red wine vinegar—17-ounce bottle
- Balsamic vinegar—17-ounce bottle
- Soy sauce (preferably reduced-sodium) or

tamari—15-ounce bottle
- Mirin (Japanese cooking wine)—17-ounce bottle

- Bay leaves—.5-ounce container
- Ground cinnamon—2.4-ounce container
- Ground allspice—2-ounce container
- Ground cloves—2-ounce container
- Ground coriander—1.6-ounce container
- Ground nutmeg—2.4-ounce container
- Ground cumin—3-ounce container
- Dried oregano—1.1-ounce container
- Cayenne—2-ounce container
- Garlic powder—2.4-ounce container
- Black peppercorns—2.4-ounce container
- Coarse-grained salt—26-ounce container

- Tabasco or hot pepper sauce (preferably made with malagueta peppers)—5-ounce bottle
- Whole-grain mustard (preferably Pommery)—12-ounce jar
- Maté tea—1 box of tea bags
- Unflavored gelatin—1-ounce box
- Shredded, unsweetened coconut—14-ounce bag
- Vanilla pod—2 pods
- Cocoa powder—12-ounce container
- Chocolate sprinkles—6-ounce container
- Brown rice (preferably Texmati or other brown basmati)—2-pound package
- Sugar—2-pound package
- Splenda—1.9-ounce box
- Whole wheat flour—2-pound package
- Cornstarch—16-pound box
- Sweetened condensed milk—14-ounce container
- Baking powder—10-ounce container
- Whole wheat wraps—1 package of 4–6 wraps
- Ovaltine—14-ounce container
- *Guaraná*—½ gallon of syrup to be mixed with water or seltzer

- White wine (Riesling, Gewürztraminer, or Portuguese *vinho verde*)—1 bottle
- Red wine (full bodied, Barolo or Burgundy)—1 bottle

- Frozen *açaí* pulp (sweetened and infused with *guaraná*)—3 packages of 4 (3.5-ounce) packets or 3 (1-pint) tubs
- Frozen acerola pulp—1 package of 4 (3.5-ounce) packets
- Frozen strawberries—16-ounce package (or same amount fresh)
- Frozen blueberries—16-ounce package (or same amount fresh)
- Frozen cut mangoes—16-ounce package (or same amount fresh)
- Frozen cut mixed fruit (berries, melon, etc.)—16-ounce package
- Frozen shrimp—16-ounce package (or same amount fresh)
- Frozen chicken stock—10-ounce container (or same amount fresh)
- Frozen vegetable stock—10-ounce container (or same amount fresh)
- Frozen broccoli—16-ounce package (or same amount fresh)
- Frozen shiitake mushrooms—16-ounce package (or same amount fresh or dried)
- Frozen edamame—10-ounce package
- Frozen phyllo dough sheets—14-ounce container

- Coconut water—4 (1-ounce) portions
- Vanilla soy milk—1 quart
- Unflavored soy milk—1 pint
- Buttermilk—1 half gallon
- Milk—1 half gallon
- Reduced-fat sour cream—8-ounce container
- Reduced-fat cream cheese—8-ounce container
- Unflavored live yogurt—8-ounce container
- *Halloumi* cheese—8-ounce container
- Emmental or Swiss cheese, sliced—10-ounce package
- Tofu—14-ounce container
- Cream (heavy or half-and-half)—1 pint
- Gnocchi (fresh)—16-ounce package

- Orange juice—1 quart
- 1 dozen eggs

- Flank steak (lean)—1 pound
- Red meat filets (buffalo, ostrich or extra-lean beef)—2 fillets
- *Chouriço*—2 sausages
- Whole chicken breast—1
- Half-chicken on the bone—1
- Sashimi-grade tuna, salmon, and mackerel—½ pound of each (buy this on Friday morning, day 20, the day of the sushi party)
- Fish head scraps—1 pound
- Dried, smoked shrimp—¼ pound

- Garlic—4 heads
- Onions—5-pound bag
- Red onion—1
- Scallions—1 bunch
- Potatoes—5-pound bag, preferably fingerling or Yukon Gold
- Sweet potato—1
- Carrots—1-pound bag
- Radishes—1 bunch
- Parsley—3 bunches
- Coriander—3 bunches
- Romaine lettuce—1 head
- Cabbage—1 small head
- Corn on the cob—2
- Watercress—5 bunches
- Arugula—1 bunch
- Spinach—1-pound bag
- Celery—1-pound bag
- Cucumber—1
- Eggplant—1, or 10 ounces of grilled slices in olive oil
- Red bell peppers—4
- Green bell peppers—3
- Yellow bell peppers—3
- Malagueta pepper—1
- Ginger—1 medium-size knob
- Tomatoes—6

- Cherry tomatoes—1 pint
- Limes—6
- Lemons—6
- Oranges—2
- Bananas—6
- Apples—3
- Pears—2

- Black-eyed peas—2 (15-ounce) cans, or 1 (16-ounce) bag dried
- Hijiki—5-ounce bag
- Roasted nori seaweed (preferably teriyaki or hot-and-spicy flavored)—.8-ounce container
- Wasabi—1-ounce tube

- Brazil nuts—1 pound
- Cashews—1 pound
- Walnuts—1 pound
- Peanuts—½ pound
- Peanut butter (crunchy or creamy)—16-ounce jar
- Pumpkin seeds—1 pound
- Pressed guava paste or *membrillo*—21-ounce package

- Palm hearts—2(14-ounce) cans
- Coconut milk—3 (14-ounce) cans
- Pumpkin—14-ounce can
- Tuna in spring water—6-ounce can
- Red miso—15-ounce container
- Pitted black gaeta olives—15-ounce container
- Sliced pickles—16-ounce jar
- Japanese pickles—7-ounce package

- Extra-virgin olive oil—34-ounce bottle
- *Dendê* oil—7-ounce bottle
- Sesame oil—6-ounce bottle
- Canola oil—32-ounce bottle
- Red wine vinegar—17-ounce bottle
- Balsamic vinegar—17-ounce bottle
- Soy sauce (preferably reduced-sodium) or tamari—15-ounce bottle
- Mirin (Japanese cooking wine)—17-ounce bottle

- Bay leaves—.5-ounce container
- Ground cinnamon—2.4-ounce container
- Ground allspice—2-ounce container
- Ground cloves—2-ounce container
- Ground coriander—1.6-ounce container
- Ground nutmeg—2.4-ounce container
- Ground cumin—3-ounce container
- Dried oregano—1.1-ounce container
- Cayenne—2-ounce container
- Garlic powder—2.4-ounce container
- Black peppercorns—2.4-ounce container
- Coarse-grained salt—26-ounce container

- Tabasco or hot pepper sauce (preferably made with malagueta peppers)—5-ounce bottle
- Whole-grain mustard (preferably Pommery)—12-ounce jar
- Maté tea—1 box of tea bags
- Unflavored gelatin—1-ounce box
- Lime-flavored gelatin—1 (3-ounce) box
- Shredded, unsweetened coconut—14-ounce bag
- Vanilla pod—2 pods
- Tapioca, organic—12-ounce container
- Brown rice (preferably Texmati or other brown basmati)—2-ounce package
- Sugar—2-ounce package
- Splenda—1.9-ounce box
- Whole wheat flour—2-pound package
- Manioc flour—16-ounce container
- Cornstarch—1-pound box
- Baking powder—10-ounce container
- Whole wheat wraps—1 package of 4–6 wraps
- Baguette, whole wheat—1
- *Guaraná*—½ gallon of syrup to be mixed with water or seltzer
- Seltzer—1 bottle

- White wine (Riesling, Gewürztraminer, or Portuguese *vinho verde*)—1 bottle

- Frozen *açaí* pulp (sweetened and infused with *guaraná*)—3 packages of 4 (3.5-ounce) packets or 3 1-pint tubs
- Frozen acerola pulp—1 package of 4 (3.5-ounce) packets
- Frozen strawberries—16-ounce package (or same amount fresh)
- Frozen blueberries—16-ounce package (or same amount fresh)
- Frozen cut mangoes—16-ounce package (or same amount fresh)
- Frozen cut mixed fruit (berries, melon, etc.)—16-ounce package
- Frozen shrimp—16-ounce package (or same amount fresh)
- Frozen chicken stock—10-ounce container (or same amount fresh)
- Frozen fish stock—10-ounce container (or same amount fresh)
- Frozen broccoli—16-ounce package (or same amount fresh)
- Frozen shiitake mushrooms—16-ounce package (or same amount fresh or dried)
- Frozen phyllo dough sheets—14-ounce container

- Coconut water—4 (11-ounce) portions
- Vanilla soy milk—1 quart
- Unflavored soy milk—1 pint
- Buttermilk—1 half gallon
- Milk—1 half gallon
- Reduced-fat sour cream—8-ounce container
- Reduced-fat cream cheese—8-ounce container
- Unflavored live yogurt—8-ounce container
- Gorgonzola cheese—8-ounce container
- Parmesan cheese—8-ounce container
- Cream (heavy or half-and-half)—1 pint
- Orange juice—1 quart
- 1 dozen eggs

- Bacon (turkey or pork)—1-pound package
- Small beef steaks (lean)—2
- Ground beef (buffalo, ostrich, or extra-lean beef)—1 pound
- *Chouriço*—2 sausages
- Whole chicken—1
- Whole turkey breast—1
- Crab meat—½ pound
- Salt cod—½ pound
- White-fleshed fish fillets (e.g., hoki, plaice, gray sole)—½ pound
- Dried, smoked shrimp—¼ pound

- Garlic—3 heads
- Onions—5-pound bag
- Red onion—1
- Scallions—1 bunch
- Potatoes—5-pound bag, preferably fingerling or Yukon Gold
- Sweet potato—1
- Carrots—1-pound bag
- Radishes—1 bunch
- Parsley—3 bunches (curly-leaf)
- Coriander—3 bunches
- Romaine lettuce—1 head
- Cabbage—1 small head
- Kale, preferably "black" or Cavolo Nero—1 bunch
- Zucchini (or other small squash)—1
- Watercress—5 bunches
- Arugula—1 bunch
- Spinach—1-pound bag
- Celery—1-pound bag
- Red bell peppers—4
- Green bell peppers—3
- Yellow bell peppers—3
- Malagueta pepper—1
- Ginger—1 medium-size knob of fresh ginger and 1 (7-ounce) packet of pickled ginger
- Tomatoes—10

- Limes—10
- Lemons—6
- Oranges—3
- Bananas—6
- Apples—3
- Pear—1

- Black-eyed peas—2 (15-ounce) cans or 1 (16-ounce) bag dried
- **Black beans—2 (15-ounce) cans, or 1 (16-ounce) bag dried**
- **Roasted nori seaweed (preferably teriyaki or hot-and-spicy flavored)—.8-ounce container**

- Brazil nuts—1 pound
- Cashews—1 pound
- Walnuts—1 pound
- Peanuts—½ pound
- Peanut butter (crunchy or creamy)—16-ounce jar
- Pumpkin seeds—1 pound
- **Pressed guava paste or *membrillo*—21-ounce package**

- **Palm hearts—14-ounce can**
- **Coconut milk—3 (14-ounce) cans**
- **Anchovy fillets packed in oil—3-ounce can**
- **Artichoke hearts in olive oil—10-ounce can**
- **Pitted black gaeta olives—15-ounce container**
- Sliced pickles—16-ounce jar
- Japanese pickles—7-ounce package
- Extra-virgin olive oil—34-ounce bottle
- *Dendê* oil—7-ounce bottle
- Sesame oil—6-ounce bottle
- Canola oil—32-ounce bottle
- Red wine vinegar—17-ounce bottle
- Balsamic vinegar—17-ounce bottle
- Soy sauce (preferably reduced-sodium) or tamari—15-ounce bottle
- Mirin (Japanese cooking wine)—17-ounce bottle

- Bay leaves—.5-ounce container
- Ground cinnamon—2.4-ounce container
- Ground allspice—2-ounce container
- Ground cloves—2-ounce container
- Ground coriander—1.6-ounce container
- Ground nutmeg—2.4-ounce container
- Ground cumin—3-ounce container
- Dried oregano—1.1-ounce container
- Cayenne—2-ounce container
- Garlic powder—2.4-ounce container
- Black peppercorns—2.4-ounce container
- Coarse-grained salt—26-ounce container

- Tabasco or hot pepper sauce (preferably made with malagueta peppers)—5-ounce bottle
- Whole-grain mustard (preferably Pommery)—12-ounce jar
- Maté tea—1 box of tea bags
- Unflavored gelatin—1-ounce box
- Shredded, unsweetened coconut—14-ounce bag
- Vanilla pod—2 pods
- **Vanilla extract—2-ounce bottle**
- **Almond extract—2-ounce bottle**
- Tapioca, organic—12-ounce container
- Brown rice (preferably Texmati or other brown basmati rice)—2-pound package
- Sugar—2-pound package
- Splenda—1.9-ounce box
- Whole wheat flour—2-pound package
- Manioc flour—16-ounce container
- Cornstarch—16-ounce box
- Baking powder—10-ounce container
- **Baking soda—1-pound box**
- **Whole wheat wraps—1 package of 4–6 wraps**
- **Baguette, whole wheat—1**
- **Panko bread crumbs—12-ounce bag**

- **White wine (Riesling, Gewürztraminer, or Portuguese *vinho verde*)—1 bottle**
- ***Cachaça*—1 bottle**
- **Brazilian rum (preferably Oronoco)—1 bottle**

- Frozen *açai* pulp (sweetened and infused with *guaraná*)—2 packages of 4 (3.5-ounce) packets, or 2 (1-pint) tubs
- Frozen acerola pulp—1 package of 4 (3.5-ounce) packets
- Frozen strawberries—16-ounce package (or same amount fresh)
- Frozen blueberries—16-ounce package (or same amount fresh)
- Frozen cut mangoes—16-ounce package (or same amount fresh)
- Frozen cut mixed fruit (berries, melon, etc.)—16-ounce package
- Frozen shrimp—16-ounce package (or same amount fresh)
- Frozen broccoli—16-ounce package (or same amount fresh)
- Frozen phyllo dough sheets—14-ounce container

- Coconut water—4 (11-ounce) portions
- Vanilla soy milk—1 quart
- Unflavored soy milk—1 pint
- Buttermilk—1 half gallon
- Milk—1 half gallon
- Reduced-fat sour cream—8-ounce container
- Reduced-fat cream cheese—8-ounce container
- Unflavored live yogurt—8-ounce container
- Grated Gruyère, Parmesan, or other cheese—8-ounce container
- Cream (heavy or half-and-half)—1 pint
- Orange juice—1 quart
- 1 dozen eggs

- Bacon (turkey or pork)—16-ounce package
- Lean beef chuck—½ pound
- Lean pork shoulder—½ pound
- Lean smoked pork shoulder—½ pound
- *Chouriço*—4 sausages
- Whole chicken—1
- Salt cod—½ pound
- Dried, smoked shrimp—¼ pound

- Garlic—3 heads
- Onions—5-pound bag
- Scallions—1 bunch
- Potatoes—5-pound bag, preferably fingerling or Yukon Gold
- Carrots—1-pound bag
- Radishes—1 bunch
- Parsley—3 bunches
- Coriander—3 bunches
- Mint—1 bunch
- Romaine lettuce—1 head
- Kale, preferably "black" or Cavolo Nero—1 bunch
- Zucchini (or other small squash)—1
- Watercress—5 bunches
- Arugula—1 bunch
- Spinach—1-pound bag
- Celery—1-pound bag
- Red bell peppers—3
- Green bell peppers—2
- Yellow bell peppers—2
- Malagueta pepper—1
- Ginger—1 medium-size knob
- Tomatoes—6
- Limes—1 dozen
- Lemons—3
- Oranges—3
- Bananas—6
- Apples—3
- Pear—1

- Black beans—2 (15-ounce) cans, or 1 (16-ounce) bag dried
- Roasted nori seaweed (preferably teriyaki or hot-and-spicy flavored)—.8-ounce container

- Brazil nuts—1 pound
- Cashews—1 pound
- Walnuts—1 pound
- Peanuts—½ pound
- Peanut butter (crunchy or creamy)—16-ounce jar

- Pumpkin seeds—1 pound
- **Pressed guava paste or *membrillo*—21-ounce package**

- **Palm hearts—2 (14-ounce) cans**
- **Coconut milk—2 (14-ounce) cans**
- **Anchovy fillets packed in oil—3-ounce can**
- **Artichoke hearts in olive oil—10-ounce can**
- **Pitted black gaeta olives—15-ounce container**
- Sliced pickles—16-ounce jar
- Japanese pickles—7-ounce package

- Extra-virgin olive oil—34-ounce bottle
- *Dendê* oil—7-ounce bottle
- Sesame oil—6-ounce bottle
- Canola oil—32-ounce bottle
- Red wine vinegar—17-ounce bottle
- Balsamic vinegar—17-ounce bottle
- Soy sauce (preferably reduced-sodium) or tamari—15-ounce bottle
- Mirin (Japanese cooking wine)—17-ounce bottle

- Bay leaves—.5-ounce container
- Ground cinnamon—2.4-ounce container
- Ground allspice—2-ounce container
- Ground cloves—2-ounce container
- Ground coriander—1.6-ounce container
- Ground nutmeg—2.4-ounce container
- Ground cumin—3-ounce container
- Dried oregano—1.1-ounce container
- Cayenne—2-ounce container
- Garlic powder—2.4-ounce container
- Black peppercorns—2.4-ounce container
- Coarse-grained salt—26-ounce container

- Tabasco or hot pepper sauce (preferably made with malagueta peppers)—5-ounce bottle
- Whole-grain mustard (preferably Pommery)—12-ounce jar
- Maté tea—1 box of tea bags
- Unflavored gelatin—1-ounce box
- Shredded, unsweetened coconut—14-ounce bag
- Vanilla pod—2 pods
- Vanilla extract—2-ounce bottle
- Almond extract—2-ounce bottle
- Tapioca, organic—12-ounce container
- **Brown rice (preferably Texmati or other brown basmati)—2-pound package**
- Sugar—2-pound package
- Splenda—1.9-ounce box
- Whole wheat flour—2-pound package
- *Pão de queijo* mix or tapioca flour (if making from scratch)—250g package premixed, or 18 ounces tapioca flour
- **Manioc flour—16-ounce container**
- Cornstarch—16-ounce box
- Baking powder—10-ounce container
- Baking soda—1-pound box
- **Whole wheat wraps—1 package of 4–6 wraps**
- **Panko bread crumbs—12-ounce bag**

- **White wine (Riesling, Gewürztraminer, or Portuguese *vinho verde*)—1 bottle**
- *Cachaça*—1 bottle
- **Brazilian rum (preferably Oronoco)—1 bottle**

MENU AND WORKOUT LOG

MONDAY

Breakfast: _____   Snacks: _____
Lunch: _____   Workout session/activity: _____
Dinner: _____

TUESDAY

Breakfast: _____   Snacks: _____
Lunch: _____   Workout session/activity: _____
Dinner: _____

WEDNESDAY

Breakfast: _____   Snacks: _____
Lunch: _____   Workout session/activity: _____
Dinner: _____

THURSDAY

Breakfast: _____   Snacks: _____
Lunch: _____   Workout session/activity: _____
Dinner: _____

FRIDAY

Breakfast: _____   Snacks: _____
Lunch: _____   Workout session/activity: _____
Dinner: _____

SATURDAY

Breakfast: _____   Snacks: _____
Lunch: _____   Workout session/activity: _____
Dinner: _____

SUNDAY

Breakfast: _____   Snacks: _____
Lunch: _____   Workout session/activity: _____
Dinner: _____

Resources

BRAZILIAN FOOD

United States

Order online from these sites to purchase *açaí* and other Amazonian fruits in frozen pulp form, *dendê* oil, *pao de queijo* mix, salt cod, *queijo de Minas* (*queijo Mineiro*), malagueta peppers, manioc flour, maté tea, *guaraná*, guava paste, and more. Make sure to compare prices!

SendexNet: www.sendexnet.com/content/v1/body.php (make sure to click on English language version if needed)
Amigo Foods: store.amigofoods.com/brazilianfood.html
Brazil Explore: www.brazilexplore.com/shop/default.aspx# (they also sell frozen goods like prepared breads, pastries, and snacks, as well as other Brazilian goods)
Brazil to Go: braziltogo.net/catalog/index.php
Sambazon: www.sambazon.com (high-quality organic frozen *açaí* and acerola pulp)
Asian Food Grocer (for Japanese staples): www.asianfoodgrocer.com
Look for Brazilian grocery stores in big cities like New York, San Francisco, Miami, Chicago, Los Angeles, and Boston. If you can't find what you're looking for online (especially Amazonian fruit pulp), you're likely to find them in these markets.
To keep your drinking water alkaline and well filtered, try the Nikken personal water filter. Go to www.nikken.com.

Europe

Finalmente Brasil (an excellent Netherlands-based supplier): www.finalmentebrasil.nl
Açaí-Café (a German-based company that sells *açaí* and other Amazonian frozen fruit pulps): www.acai-cafe.com/ACAI_cafe_german/index_german.htm

CAPOEIRA INFORMATION

Capoeira.com: www.capoeira.com
Capoeirista.com: www.capoeirista.com
Arte Capoeira: www.artecapoeira.com

PILATES INFORMATION

The Pilates Method Alliance: www.Pilatesmethodalliance.com
Classical Pilates Technique: The Complete Mat Workout Series DVD, available at www.amazon.com

BRAZILIAN TOURISM

Brazil Tour (Ministry of Tourism): www.braziltour.com/site/en/home/index.php
Pedro Müller Starpoint Surf School: www.escolapedromuller.com.br
Ipanema Sport Club: www.ipanemasportclub.com.br

BRAZILIAN MUSIC

Bossa Nova.fm: www.bossanova.fm (a very comprehensive blog and site with excellent pod-
    casts)
All Brazilian Music Guide: www.allbrazilianmusic.com (perhaps the most complete and com-
    prehensive online guide)

BRAZILIAN FOOTBALL

Futebol, the Brazilian Way of Life: www.futebolthebrazilianwayoflife.com (the very informative
    and entertaining blog by Alex Bellos, author of the book *Futebol: The Brazilian Way of Life*)
Samba Foot: www.sambafoot.com/en (Web site in English, French, and Portuguese)

BRAZILIAN FASHION

Havaianas US: www.havaianasus.com (the ultimate in flip-flops)
Rosa Cha: rosacha.com.br (chic bikini wear by Brazilian designer Amir Slama)
Florida Brasil: www.floridabrasil.com/english/produtos.html (carries bikinis, flip-flops, and
    more)

Bibliography

Bassoul, Eliane. *Em Paz Com a Mesa: 32 variações sobre um só Tema: alimentação*. Rio de Janeiro, Brazil: Vieira e Lent, 2004.

Capoeira, Nestor. *The Little Capoeira Book*. Berkeley, California: North Atlantic Books, 1995, 2003.

Castro, Ruy. *Rio de Janeiro: Carnival Under Fire*. London: Bloomsbury Publishing, 2004.

Gil, Felippe. *Frutas: Sabor à Primeira Dentada*. São Paulo, Brazil: Editora Senac, 2004.

Levine, Robert M. *Brazilian Legacies*. Armonk, New York: M. E. Sharpe, 1997.

Page, Joseph A. *The Brazilians*. Boston, Massachusetts: Addison Wesley Publishing Company, 1996.

Pessanha, Luciana. *Gula Gula: Comida Bossa Nova*. São Paulo, Brazil: Editora Senac, 2002.

Reader's Digest, eds. *Coma Bem, Vive Melhor: Super Saladas*. São Paulo: Reader's Digest Brasil LTDA, 2004.

Silva, Silvestre, and Helena Tassara. *Frutas Brasil Frutas*. São Paulo, Brazil: Empresa das Artes, 2005.

Acknowledgments

This book would have remained just another grand-idea-gone-unexecuted without the help of numerous friends and colleagues who supported me and the project throughout its twists and turns.

All at St. Martin's Press and my editor, Sheila Curry Oakes, deserve thanks for allowing me to make this book. At my very first meeting with them, I was made to feel as if this book was a winner—which, apart from a nice ego massage, focused my concentration. I am so grateful for their support.

Jeremy Katz, my agent at Sanford J. Greenburger Associates, deserves kudos and earns my eternal respect for having had the courage to take me and the book on. Moreover, he went a step further and aggressively streamlined my prose and ideas—an invaluable asset. For me, he will always be a superlative editor in agent's guise. I'd also like to thank Teri Tobias for her support and efforts on the international front.

The team who helped me produce this book both in New York and Brazil equally share in whatever accolades the Brazilian Bikini Body Program brand accrues. I could not have done it without them. First, thanks go to those who shot and worked on the photos: Carlos Emilio de Sá e Silva, Marco Antonio Guimarães, Arthur Cohen, and Marina Grau. I'd especially like to praise Eliane Lazzaris for her fantastic graphic work, and I can't imagine doing anything without the help and encouragement from my dear friend Richard Ng, who always comes through in a pinch for me—and did, over and over again. A hearty *obrigado* to Marco Pederneira and Diogo Schmidt of the Ipanema Sport Club in Rio, for magnanimously allowing us to use their lovely gym. And I must reserve a special gesture of enormous gratitude for the beautiful and patient models: Carolina Nakamura and Guilherme Licurgo, both with 40 Graus of Rio de Janeiro. Carolina and Guilherme are as generous as they are hot, and I fervently hope that this book will propel them to the heights they both deserve.

In supporting this book, I could have no friendlier assistance than I had from Vicente Bastos Ribeiro, Pedro Müller, and Leandro Carvalho; all my colleagues at Equinox Fitness Clubs; Fred Bootsma and Henry Obadiah, financial whizzes extraordinaire on opposite sides of the Atlantic; and David McLoughlin, a man of redoubtable musical knowledge and kindness.

I owe a very deep debt of gratitude to all my wonderful teachers who have helped me to develop my knowledge over so many years: In particular, I want to thank Bob Liekens, whose passionate insistence on precision has been a constant source of inspiration for over a decade; and the incredibly powerful capoeira teachers Mestre Mucuíu and Mestre Edna Lima in New York. What very little I really know about capoeira, I owe it all to them.

Of course, this book could not have existed without my family: Patricia, Maria Alice, and Elio; Clara, Roger, and Nice; Marcio and Miguel; Ralph and Leda; Isabel and Adriana. How else could I have come up with this concept without having been a part of their stories, their food, their recipes, their adventures, and their lives?

To all the kind friends who contributed actively to this project, a big hug from me: Alan Archment; Ted Allen and Barry Rice (whose assistance at critical moments in Brazil and in New York provided support for which I will always be grateful); Laura Aswad; Ji Baek; Dr. Maurice Beer; Bryan Bradley; Marcel Brouns; Abhi Chaki and Shamma Fidaly; Mara Flynn; Richard, Anita, and Zoe Gottehrer; Jay Hirschson; Elizabeth Holland; Ian Kerner; Joon Ma; Monica Mello; Shazna Nessa; Greg Posey and Lex Kranendonk; David Sack; Eric Swenson; Brenda and Ezequiel Szafir-Holcman; Justin Teodoro; Nancy Wong; and Gabriel Zichermann.

Finally, I get down on my knees and thank Jerry and Helene Spiegel and their family, without whom this book would simply have never happened.

Index